NAVIGATING THE DEMENTIA JOURNEY

A COMPASSIONATE GUIDE TO UNDERSTANDING, SUPPORTING, AND LIVING WITH DEMENTIA

JEFF HOLLITZ

BRICKTOP PUBLISHING

© **Copyright 2023 - All rights reserved.**

The content contained within this book may not be reproduced, duplicated or transmitted without direct written permission from the author or the publisher.

Under no circumstances will any blame or legal responsibility be held against the publisher, or author, for any damages, reparation, or monetary loss due to the information contained within this book, either directly or indirectly.

Legal Notice:

This book is copyright protected. It is only for personal use. You cannot amend, distribute, sell, use, quote or paraphrase any part, or the content within this book, without the consent of the author or publisher.

Disclaimer Notice:

Please note the information contained within this document is for educational and entertainment purposes only. All effort has been executed to present accurate, up to date, reliable, complete information. No warranties of any kind are declared or implied. Readers acknowledge that the author is not engaged in the rendering of legal, financial, medical or professional advice. The content within this book has been derived from various sources. Please consult a licensed professional before attempting any techniques outlined in this book.

By reading this document, the reader agrees that under no circumstances is the author responsible for any losses, direct or indirect, that are incurred as a result of the use of the information contained within this document, including, but not limited to, errors, omissions, or inaccuracies.

CONTENTS

Introduction — 5

1. DELVING INTO THE MIND OF A DEMENTIA PATIENT — 17
   - Brief Description of a Dementia Patient — 19
   - The Effect of Dementia on the Brain — 21
   - Summary — 29

2. DISSECTING DEMENTIA: THE SILENT THIEF — 31
   - Dementia Defined — 32
   - Causes and Risk Factors of Dementia — 33
   - Symptoms of Dementia — 38
   - Summary — 41

3. DISCOVERING THE MANY FACES OF DEMENTIA — 45
   - Types of Dementia — 46
   - Stages of Dementia — 53
   - Summary — 60

4. IDENTIFYING THE IMPACT OF DEMENTIA — 63
   - Effects of Dementia on the Person With the Condition — 64
   - Effects of Dementia on a Person's Loved Ones or Caregivers — 67
   - Effects of Dementia on a Person's Relationship With Loved Ones — 70
   - Summary — 74

5. BREAKING DOWN BARRIERS — 77
   - Communication and Dementia: A Review — 78
   - Verbal Communication — 82
   - Non-Verbal Communication — 84
   - Other Tips — 86

What Not to Do	87
Summary	89
6. DEALING WITH A FADING MEMORY	91
Dementia and Memory Loss: A Review	92
How to Help Your Loved One Cope With Memory Loss	93
Brain Exercises	100
Summary	102
7. RESPONDING TO TROUBLING BEHAVIOR	105
Dementia and Changes in Behavior: A Review	106
General Tips: Follow the P.E.E.L Method	108
Specific Tips for the Most Common Behavior Changes	111
Summary	117
8. IMPROVING DAILY LIFE AMID DEMENTIA	121
Personal Hygiene	123
Nutrition	126
Exercise	130
Summary	134
9. STRENGTHENING YOUR BOND	137
What to Consider When Coming up With Activities for Your Loved One	138
Suggested Activities	140
Summary	147
10. TAKING CARE OF YOURSELF	149
What Is Caregiver Burnout?	150
Symptoms of Caregiver Burnout	151
Tips to Manage Caregiver Burnout	152
Summary	159
Conclusion	161
References	165

INTRODUCTION

To care for those who once cared for us is one of the highest honors.

— TIA WALKER

Did you know globally, approximately 55 million people are living with dementia? This statistic increases every year, with almost 10 million newly diagnosed people with dementia worldwide (World Health Organization [WHO], 2023). Dementia is a neurodegenerative disorder caused by various illnesses and injuries to the brain that affect memory, problem-solving, and other cognitive abilities, emotion, and behavior. Of the various forms of dementia, Alzheimer's disease is the most prevalent type of dementia. Of all dementia cases, about 60 to 70 percent of them are Alzheimer's disease. Currently, amongst the elderly, dementia is the seventh most common cause of death and one of the biggest causes of disability and dependency worldwide. Unfortunately, this results in those affected needing care and assistance in everyday activities. Common early symptoms of dementia include but are not limited to the following:

- Memory loss,
- Struggles with performing tasks they usually do,
- Difficulty with language and communication, and
- Fluctuations in their personality.

Furthermore, the medical research and science fields have not discovered a cure for dementia yet. The number of people living with dementia around the world will rise to 139 million by 2050 and is likely to be even higher in low- and middle-income countries (Alzheimer's Disease International [ADI], n.d.a). The number of people affected in any country, city, town, or place rises every three seconds. The statistics on the number of people who have not received a diagnosis are alarming. Of those people living with dementia, 75 percent of them worldwide have not received a formal diagnosis. The worldwide cost of undiagnosed cases of dementia is estimated to be $1.3 trillion.

Many famous personalities have suffered from dementia in different fields of work, such as entertainment, sports, and politics. Below is a list of 5 people in each category: Actors and actresses, sportsmen and women, authors, and other public figures you may be unaware were formally diagnosed with dementia.

Actors

- Burgess Meredith, actor (November 16, 1907 - September 9, 1997)
- Sean Connery, actor (August 25, 1930 - October 31, 2020)
- Evelyn Keyes, actress (November 20, 1916 - July 4, 2008)
- Robin Williams, actor (July 21, 1951 - August 11, 2014)
- Joanne Woodward, actress (February 27, 1930 - present)

Athletes

- Marvin James Owen, baseball player (March 22, 1906 - June 22, 1991)
- Betty Schwartz, track player (August 23, 1911 - May 18, 1999)
- Sugar Ray Robinson, boxer (May 3, 1921 - April 12, 1989)

- Bill Quackenbush, hockey player (March 2, 1922 - September 12, 1999)
- Pat Summitt, basketball trainer (June 14, 1952 - June 27, 2016)

Authors

- Ben Bradlee, journalist and newspaper editor (August 26, 1921 - October 21, 2014)
- Iris Murdoch, writer, and philosopher (July 15, 1919 - February 8, 1999)
- Pauline Phillips, Dear Abby advice columnist (July 4, 1918 - January 16, 2013)
- Alfred van Vogt, science fiction writer (April 26, 1912 - January 26, 2000)
- Elwyn Brooks White, author (July 11, 1899 - October 1, 1985)

Politicians and changemakers

- Raul Silva Henriquez, a Roman Catholic cardinal and defender of human rights (September 27, 1907 - April 9, 1999)
- Rosa Parks, activist in the American civil rights movement (February 4, 1913 - October 24, 2005)
- Ronald Reagan, 40th President of the United States of America (USA) (February 6, 1911 - June 5, 2004)

- Margaret Thatcher, Europe's first female prime minister (October 13, 1925 - April 8, 2013)
- Harold Wilson, Europe's prime minister (March 11, 1916 - May 24, 1995)

One of the most-known celebrities diagnosed with dementia was actress Rita Hayworth, who rose to fame in the 1940s (Long Island Alzheimer's and Dementia Center, 2021). She battled with Alzheimer's for over a decade before being formally diagnosed in 1980 and passing away in 1987. At that time, most of the public knew little about the neurodegenerative disorder, and her death helped raise public awareness of Alzheimer's disease. She was taken care of by her daughter, Princess Yasmin Aga Khan, who became a candid philanthropist of the illness. She serves on the Board of Directors as the vice chairperson for the Alzheimer's and Related Disorders Association and the President of Alzheimer's Disease International, an amalgamation of Alzheimer's associations worldwide (Leung, 2019).

Robin Williams was an actor who started his career in the entertainment industry in America in the 1970s as a stand-up comedian. His breakout role was in the Mork & Mindy television series in the late 1970s. He was an award-winning actor. During his career, he was awarded an Academy Award for Best Supporting Actor in the movie Good Will Hunting and won 6 Golden Globe Awards and 5 Grammy Awards. Many people were shocked when he passed away in 2014. The autopsy results revealed that he suffered from Lewy body Dementia, a progressive brain disorder that has similar symptoms to other neurodegenerative diseases such as Parkinson's and Alzheimer's disease. His surviving wife, Susan Williams, believed that this condition caused her late husband to experience poor mental health and ultimately was the cause of his death and not the rumors in the media that alcohol and drug use were the results of his death (Long Island Alzheimer's and Dementia Center, 2021; 2023).

Ronald Reagan was an actor in Hollywood who later in life was appointed as the 33rd Governor of California and the 40th president of the United States despite all odds stacked against him (Long Island Alzheimer's and Dementia Center, 2021). During his political career, he had the nickname "Great Communicator" because he was a charismatic and charming speaker who captured audiences' attention. He was elected for a second term in office as President, which many believed was due to his positive outlook on the future of America. His most well-known quote is, "Mr. Gorbachev, tear down this wall!" which goes down in the history of America as an all-time turning point in getting the Berlin Wall in Germany to fall. When his political career ended, he went on to live a modest life in California and was formally diagnosed with Alzheimer's disease at 83 years old. Similar to Rita, Ronald battled with Alzheimer's disease for a decade and succumbed to his death at 93 years old as a result of pneumonia.

Nowadays, many helpful resources are available online, and organizations can provide information and a range of support to people living with dementia and their carers. Finding an organization or association near your home can help you get advice on mental health services and care facilities that are available near you and answer your questions (ADI, n.d.a). It can be one of the most life-saving decisions that a carer can take to protect and support their mental health because approximately more than 50 percent of carers around the world have acknowledged that their health and mental health have been negatively affected even though they feel fulfilled with performing their role (ADI, n.d.a).

Despite the availability of information and resources about dementia, it is normal to feel you may not know enough about this condition and how it will affect your loved one as the disease progresses. Nothing is wrong with fear and worry about what might happen from the early to late stages of the condition. Also, fear can creep in when you do not want to let your loved one living with dementia down, especially when you are their primary caregiver. Many carers worry that they might fail to provide the necessary care that their loved one needs. That can make one feel as though they are inadequate, not doing a good enough job, and others can struggle with accepting they might need help.

Experiencing guilt about feeling frustrated and tired of dealing with your loved one living with dementia is something that can happen. Some carers can feel guilty whenever they get irritable or even angry at their loved one living with dementia, especially during difficult times, such as when the dementia symptoms manifest. If you have a partner and children, you could feel guilty about dividing your attention between your loved one with dementia and your partner and children.

Even though it is beyond the carer and their loved one's control, feeling frustrated when faced with dementia symptoms is common. Normal daily activities, such as dressing, bathing, and eating, may become sources of deep frustration for them. Behaviors often associated with dementia, such as wandering or repeatedly asking questions, can frustrate carers.

Feeling drained physically, emotionally, mentally, and financially from the stress of caring for someone with dementia comes with the responsibility, since carers spend most of their time in their role and tend to neglect their needs. Often, the demands of this role are overwhelming and can cause anyone to experience fatigue. Worrying that you could experience burnout if things do not improve soon is normal.

Also, another consequence for carers who spend most of their time taking care of their loved ones with dementia is that they have limited time to have a social life, meaning they can find that they rarely go out to see their friends, talk to other loved ones or interact with other people.

Before considering writing this book, I wondered if other people had similar experiences and feelings to my story. Like most people in my generation, my parents never sat down during dinner to discuss anything related to health issues. Never. When my grandparents began to deteriorate cognitively, I was only told, "It is just old age," and that is all I knew about dementia. I also noticed that everyone in my genetic family tree lived to old age but suffered from "just old age."

My grandfather had Alzheimer's disease, and he would exhibit aggressive behavior, including violent outbursts that were difficult to understand why he was reacting that way in non-violent situations. The day before he passed, I remember he uttered my name, smiled, and disappeared again. His disappearing act was not shocking, but the facility staff was shocked when he remembered my name because he had difficulty remembering anyone or anything.

Also, it was baffling that he remembered my name when he looked and smiled at me because he had not seen me in over a decade. My other grandfather would change subjects midsentence while conversing with you. I found that to be highly frustrating during conversations, even though I initially did not realize it. As time went on and his symptoms of dementia got progressively worse, my confusion even worsened too.

At this time in my life, my mother was living in an assisted facility. I could not care for her any longer because I became overwhelmed. Conversations with my mother were seemingly smooth, but in five minutes, it felt like she scrambled all the details; I did not know what was true or mixed up thinking. To me, it seemed as though she was saying random sentences, such as "the time when I threw a rock across the road …", and "how the neighbor's boy was [in] trouble …". At first, I expected her to share more of the story; I thought it would be like a fun recollection. Nonetheless, that never happened. She could only put together those simple sentences to retell the story.

I inevitably got frustrated. I am not proud of what I am about to share; however, after getting into emotional fights with my mother, I decided I should have her admitted to an assisted living facility. I vividly remember my mother telling the nurse I had taken her money. I got mildly angry. I understood that getting memories mixed up would often happen, but telling absolute untruths about me was shocking. In my mind, I could not understand why she would be telling lies to people about the person who spent significant time and resources caring for her. However, after focusing my energy and time on healing and researching dementia, I understood why I struggled and failed at dealing with her "old age." Also, I got to forgive myself when I started engaging in research for this book.

I learned things I never knew and was never taught. I understood the pain and confusion the dementia patient and caregiver experience daily. Toward finishing my research, I accepted that it is most likely that I might live to "old age" and suffer from cognitive deterioration. I also have the opportunity to share the knowledge I have gained to teach my children, nieces, and nephews about dementia so that they will understand how to notice the early symptoms, deal with it and find support to help them and their family members suffering from the disease.

I have been helping individuals and families who have a loved one with dementia cope with the condition. My experiences, research, and discussions with others in the same situation have also helped me develop the proper techniques and approaches when dealing with a loved one with dementia. I know the struggles of someone who has to witness a loved one deteriorate because of dementia. I hope that by sharing my knowledge and learnings, relationships do not have to suffer, and both you and your loved ones benefit from an improved quality of life even while dealing with dementia.

Most books about dementia only discuss the condition, including the symptoms and causes, and the ones suffering from it but do not tackle how it also affects others. In this book, you will get tips on how to effectively communicate with your loved ones with dementia, how to deal with symptoms such as memory loss and behavioral changes, and what to expect daily. You will also learn the importance of caring for yourself to care for your loved one with dementia effectively. This book serves as an ultimate roadmap for those struggling to meet the needs of their loved ones with dementia. It offers easy-to-follow steps to help you care for your loved one and yourself. It took me between 3 and 4 years to accumulate the knowledge shared in this book.

Those who take care of people with dementia are often referred to as "invisible patients" because of the adverse impact of the condition on them as well. By reading this book, you will gain a deeper understanding of dementia, those who suffer from it, and their roles as caregivers and support systems. As a result, they would find it more manageable to deal with their loved one who has dementia with compassion, patience, grace, an openness to change, and love every day.

After reading this book, hopefully, you will feel equipped with valuable information about the condition and know how to deal with it properly. You will have renewed hope, a new perspective, and the right attitude to care for your loved one living with dementia, no matter how difficult it gets. Also, hopefully, you will learn how to adequately navigate caring for your loved one living with dementia, especially in terms of communication, coping with memory loss, emotional and behavioral changes, and managing daily living.

In the next chapter, you will explore what happens inside the mind of an individual suffering from dementia, specifically how it damages and affects their brain functions.

1

DELVING INTO THE MIND OF A DEMENTIA PATIENT

The mystery of what goes on inside the mind of another person becomes terrifyingly impenetrable in the final stages of dementia; twilight to pitch dark at the vanishing line between life and death.

— NICCI GERRARD

There are so many fascinating facts about the human brain. Perhaps how the brain functions could arguably be the most interesting fact. Do you enjoy reading books, magazines, or your local newspaper? Have you ever read a series of several books, such as the *Bridgerton* series? When we read a book, our brains interpret the text of letters in a *Bridgerton* book as words and cultivate those words into an interesting story that captivates your attention and stays in your memory. Then, it puts together those memories of reading those first installments of the book series into a great adventure. Thus, the entire book series is a thrilling adventure from the first installment to the last.

Beyond reading, comprehension, and remembering, your brain helps you organize, plan, make decisions, and recognize people, animals, and places, such as cities, towns, landmarks, etc. Also, your brain controls your bodily movements and any activity you do voluntarily or involuntarily, such as breathing, circulating blood, and heartbeat.

Do you know where your brain gets its power? There are 100 billion nerve cells that give your brain the ability to enable you to read, think, remember, plan, decide, move your body, and do other activities (Alzheimer's Association, 2023a). Each nerve cell in your body communicates with one another through 100 microscopic connections that neuroscientists call synapses. These tiny connections create webs of neurons that are arguably more complex than the networks of a computer.

In these microscopic connections, the nerve cells in your brain share information using small electrical signals and vibrations of unique messenger chemicals. Your brain identifies everything you have ever known in repetitive sequences of nerve cells clustered into networks and the strength of the signals from one cell to another. When you learn anything new, your brain creates a unique sequence of networks, and specific signals become more robust than others.

Every moment in your wake and sleep, millions of messages shoot throughout your nerve cell networks allowing your brain to accept, compute and store information and send directives across the whole body (Alzheimer's Association, 2023a).

BRIEF DESCRIPTION OF A DEMENTIA PATIENT

When caring for a person with dementia, you will see them change progressively over time. No one can prepare you to manage to see your loved one deteriorate. Feeling powerless is normal because there is nothing you can do besides making the changes that are happening to your loved one to occur in peace. Also, these changes are not your fault or anybody else, and no one can stop them from happening to your loved one. The changes are a result of the person's brain not working as it used to.

No doctor can confidently know what changes someone with dementia will be because every person diagnosed with dementia is different. You can get people with dementia who forget details, such as your name, phone number, physical address, first graduation, or birthday. They can find it challenging to speak to you coherently, or they might act strangely, which can cause you to feel confused and even frustrated. Some people with dementia have problems with their vision and might get scared or angry about not seeing things correctly.

It is rare to find dementia patients who suffer from the same problems simultaneously. Some people with dementia can change slowly over months or years.

Below are descriptions of what dementia looks like from the perspectives of their loved ones (Alzheimer's Research, 2023):

- "My grandmother had difficulties with her speech; she could not speak to any of us anymore like she used to. It seemed she knew what she wanted to say but could not get her words out."
- "He is always disoriented. For instance, I will return from the supermarket and notice he has moved things to random spots in the house and sometimes he leaves the house and goes to places very far."
- "When I would go see her, I would see her lying in bed at her care home, and she would be unable to do anything for herself. She would not eat and felt so exhausted. That would break my heart."
- "She would open all the kitchen drawers and take out items with contents inside them. She would empty each item's contents onto the kitchen countertop."
- "He does not remember anyone besides his brother, my grandfather, and calls him dad."

- "She always fails to remember me and our family members."
- "We usually enjoy a six-course meal every night at dinner. She cannot tell whether she is hungry and does not recall if she has already had something to eat."
- "He always asks the same questions repeatedly. It can be annoying and it feels like my patience is getting tested."
- "We were worried and fearful about him possibly getting lost."
- "When she goes to the shops, she always buys the same item twice."
- "She enjoys having a couple of drinks after dinner and then fails to remember that she has already had some drinks and ends up drinking some more."
- "If she is looking for something, she tends to forget what she was looking for and then gets upset with us all of a sudden."

THE EFFECT OF DEMENTIA ON THE BRAIN

Dementia affects both the brain and the patient diagnosed with it. Thus, it is crucial to understand how your brain operates.

The Importance of Neurons

As mentioned earlier, our brain has tens of billions of nerve cells that process and send out information via electrical and chemical signals (Vera, 2023). Your brain progressively gets smaller to some extent as you get older than when you are younger, but you do not lose neurons. Dementia negatively affects the brain by causing damage to the neurons. Similar to Alzheimer's disease, with dementia, the neurons stop working normally and lose connection with one another and begin to disintegrate until they die out.

When neurons are not performing as they should, certain areas in the brain begin to suffer and get impaired. Communication and repair centers are one of the first aspects of the brain that get affected. Also, other aspects of the brain that get affected are the areas of the brain that control memory functions, such as the hippocampus.

As time passes, the cerebral cortex will begin to get impaired, and this causes someone diagnosed with dementia to experience problems with language, thinking, and social interactions (Vera, 2023).

Areas of the Brain Affected by Dementia

To understand the areas of the brain affected by dementia, it is essential for someone who thinks they might have dementia to see a neurologist for a thorough assessment (Crystal Run Healthcare, 2019). That will determine the various factors leading to the number of nerve cells dying and will specifically identify the areas of the brain that are negatively impacted by neuron loss and tissue damage. Once you get a more in-depth assessment, you should investigate the specific functional symptoms that can show which brain lobes are involved.

Frontal Lobe Involvement

The brain's frontal lobe functions consist of organization, planning, and controlling socially undesirable behavior. When a person gets their frontal lobe attacked with Alzheimer's disease or dementia, the patient can experience difficulties with managing the following symptoms (Crystal Run Healthcare, 2019):

- Feeling demotivated or losing interest in activities,
- Feeling tired, lethargic, and sleepy,
- Engaging in the same behavior that is not useful or helpful in any way, such as opening and closing the cupboards or wiping plates from the cupboards for no reason, and
- Engaging in unusual or socially undesirable behavior, for example, being aggressive, using expletives, taking off their clothes, eating items unsuitable for human consumption, uncontrolled sexual behavior, or defecating in front of people.

Temporal Lobe Involvement

The temporal lobe plays a significant role in memory, particularly the episodic memory. Encoding new information in our brains and retrieving it from our memory later, when needed, is possible because the temporal lobe controls the act of taking in new information and recalling when Mother's Day will be this year. Alzheimer's disease and dementia usually cause damage to the temporal lobes of the brain. That can make it difficult for someone with these neurodegenerative diseases to store and remember something that happened recently.

When someone with Alzheimer's disease or dementia is experiencing the early symptoms of memory loss, using visual cues, such as photographs, or verbal cues, such as phrases, can help to trigger the retrieval of events that have already happened. Patients with Alzheimer's commonly store semantic memory more quickly than episodic memory, as they can remember how to speak or perform a meaningful task, such as making tacos using their grandmother's favorite recipe. However, since they struggle with retaining episodic memory, it is difficult to recall the people and events surrounding the time they had their grandmother's tacos for dinner to celebrate something.

Parietal Lobe Involvement

The functions of the parietal lobes are to interpret sensory information. It is essential for analyzing different facial expressions and recognizing people's faces. When a patient has their parietal lobes damaged as a result of the progress of the disease, they may lose one or more of the following abilities (Crystal Run Healthcare, 2019):

- Performing basic mathematical reasoning.
- Reading and comprehending instructions.
- Knowing the difference between left and right.
- Writing clearly or in a logically.
- Drawing illustrations, making sketches or paintings.
- Identifying faces, places, or items (i.e., visual agnosia).
- Finding and picking up objects (i.e., constructional apraxia).

Occipital Lobe Involvement

The occipital lobes process visual input and help us understand what we look at daily. It is one brain area that hardly ever gets impaired by Alzheimer's disease. However, if Alzheimer's disease impairs it, the patient may start seeing things that are not there or have difficulty recognizing household items that they are familiar with and inappropriately use them.

Different Ways Dementia Affects the Brain

Plaques and Tangles

Alzheimer's disease causes beta-amyloid proteins and neurofibrillary tangles to constrict normal functioning nerve cells (Vera, 2023). The beta-amyloid proteins and neurofibrillary tangles can create problems with cell functioning and disrupt the communication and pathways of the neuron's system. When the ability of the neurons to share information is disrupted and blocked, that can affect memory and cell renewal.

Chronic Inflammation

Rather than helping to prevent the brain from developing debris, chronic inflammation can form from accumulating glial cells. They result in causing damage to healthy neurons instead of shielding those healthy neurons.

Vascular Disorders

An example of a vascular disorder is a stroke, which can considerably decrease blood flow and oxygen to the person's brain. Also, it can cause the blood-brain barrier to disintegrate substantially to the extent that the brain is unprotected from harmful agents.

Loss of Neural Connections and Cell Death

As time passes, healthy nerve cells get impaired, and the likelihood of cell death across the entire brain increases. The interconnectedness between the different neurons may fail and never go through the cell renewal process. When a dementia patient gets to the last stages, their brain gradually declines. That can cause a significant loss of brain volume (Vera, 2023).

Neuroscientist Dr. Barbara Lipska suffered from dementia in late adulthood (CarePredict, 2018). At first, she experienced her hand disappearing in front of her face. She thought this might have been the result of a brain tumor. For most of her life, she dedicated herself to studying abnormalities in rodents and human brains as director of the human brain bank at the National Institute of Mental Health.

Her inkling about a brain tumor as the cause of her disease was correct. Numerous melanoma tumors developed in her prefrontal cortex, and 18 tumors would continue to grow during her treatment. When she lost sight of her hand in front of her face, that moment saw her undergo a series of experimental treatments involving surgeries, radiation, and an immunotherapy clinical trial. Despite these medical treatments, Barbara went on to experience severe brain swelling that put pressure on the prefrontal cortex. As a result, she experienced many common cognitive changes in dementia patients.

It is rare to find a dementia patient who can share their living experience with this condition and their recovery journey. You can read more about it in detail in her novel *The Neuroscientist Who Lost Her Mind.*

The shortened version of her experience is that she could not recognize that she had dementia despite being well-trained in the symptoms. To her, it felt as though the world, people, and even her neighborhood had changed, not her perception. The part of her brain responsible for communicating when something was wrong was impaired. Barbara was more concerned and anxious about people's judgment and changes in her ability to do things herself and routine instead of the fear of cognitive decline over time because of the progression of the disease.

Barbara experienced confusion in recognizing objects and places. She would find herself lost in her neighborhood or on paths she knew well. She would wonder why things got moved to a different location or who moved them, and this would cause her to mistrust her loved ones.

Before her brain swelled, she had a solid and assertive personality. After her brain swelled, she became irritable, impatient, impulsive, and did not feel the need to bond with her family. The people around her noticed changes in her personality and asked the doctor for a scan, and later on, she got confirmation that she had significant swelling in her brain. Her friends, family, and doctor's insight proved vital for her recovery.

With her irritability, Barbara could not recognize her body's needs, such as eating when she feels hungry and going to bed when she feels tired. Also, she suffered from an inability to plan to meet her body's needs, and when she would get angry at a person, a place, or about an event, she would focus on addressing those issues. Even though her family would offer to help her, it felt as though, from her perspective, they were getting in the way of solving the problem. Also, she had a significantly large body-budget and could not spare the time and energy to hear their solutions to her problems (CarePredict, 2018).

SUMMARY

- The human brain has 100 billion neurons that communicate with each other at 100 trillion connections using electrical signals and chemicals that allow your brain to receive, interpret and retain input and send instructions to the rest of your body.
- Dementia, from the perspective of a loved one, is experienced from an outsider's stance and feelings of frustration, confusion, anxiety, and concern for their loved one with dementia.
- Dementia affects the brain by damaging healthy neurons as it causes them to stop functioning normally.
- As the disease progresses, other parts of the brain get affected, such as the frontal, temporal, parietal, and occipital lobes.
- Dementia impacts the brain in different ways, such as developing plaques and tangles around nerve cells that block the normal functioning and

communication of neurons. Also, it causes chronic inflammation that damages the nerve cells. Dementia can give rise to vascular disorders that impair the blood-brain barrier. Over time, patients will experience neuron loss and cell death, and in the late stages of the disease, their brain atrophies, which causes a significant loss of brain volume.
- Dr. Barbara Lipska, a neuroscientist, tells her story of suffering from dementia in late adulthood, which began due to a brain tumor, and her family, friends, and doctor helped her recover.

In the next chapter, you will explore the condition in-depth and understand the general causes and symptoms. Some people describe dementia as a slow and sneaky condition that robs people of their identity, memories, and independence. As such, it is often referred to by many as a "silent thief," and many people dread and fear it.

2

DISSECTING DEMENTIA: THE SILENT THIEF

For a couple of minutes, imagine you are having lunch in the care facility with your father. You find him looking at you with a vacant gaze as though he does not recognize you or even know who you are. However, you visit him weekly because you love him and feel like it is your duty as his son. In your mind, you battle with the decision: Do you commit to spending time with someone who does not remember who you are even though he is your father? Or do you instead commit to spending time with your children?

Have you ever heard people referring to dementia as the "silent thief"? Dementia is regarded as a "silent thief" because when it penetrates the brain cells of a dementia patient, it slowly takes away their memories without them knowing about it (Az, 2017). When days and weeks go by with a vague or no recollection of what happened, then years seem like they have gone with the dust. Depending on the severity of Alzheimer's disease, patients will have difficulty planning for and looking forward to their future. And then, they will gradually stop remembering their past. When that happens, it is nearly impossible to control this damage.

DEMENTIA DEFINED

Many definitions of dementia exist in the science and medical fields. Simply put, dementia is not a single disease. Instead, it is a syndrome, a cluster of symptoms caused by other underlying medical conditions that lead to dementia (WebMD, 2023).

Some definitions from research institutions like the World Health Organization (2023) and the Centers for Disease Control and Prevention (2019) will expand on that definition by stating that dementia is a condition that has many symptoms that become chronic or progressively worsen with time, leading to cognitive decline, which is unusual to the typical effects of aging. This cognitive decline can affect a person's ability to think, remember, organize, plan, and perform everyday activities.

Other non-academic sources explain that dementia is a mental disorder that may impair two or more brain functions, such as memory, focus, attention, reasoning, language, emotions, judgment, and behavior (Leonard, 2022). These cognitive impairments can severely affect a person's daily, social or occupational functioning (WedMD, 2023).

Hopefully, with these definitions, you will use them to formulate your definition that you will remember and apply to your situation.

CAUSES AND RISK FACTORS OF DEMENTIA

Dementia has several causes that result from various diseases and injuries that primarily or secondarily affect the brain, such as Alzheimer's disease or stroke.

Causes of Dementia

Below is a list of some of the common causes of dementia:

- **Neurodegenerative diseases**: "Neurodegenerative" describes neurons that slowly stop functioning or do not function normally and, over time, die (Leonard, 2022). As mentioned earlier, the synapses, the connections between the neurons, are how the neurons share information across the different brain areas. When there is a miscommunication between the neuron-to-neuron links, that can cause mental dysfunction. Examples of this cognitive dysfunction in the synapses include Alzheimer's, Parkinson's disease with dementia, vascular dementia, and chronic alcohol use disorder.

Another cause is the heterogeneous clinical syndrome known as frontotemporal lobar degeneration. It is an umbrella term for a wide range of medical conditions associated with degenerating the frontal and temporal lobes. This type of degeneration includes frontotemporal dementia, Pick's disease, supranuclear palsy, and corticobasal degeneration.

- **Structural brain disorders**: These include normal pressure hydrocephalus and subdural hematoma.
- **Metabolic disorders**: These include hypothyroidism, vitamin B12 deficiency, and kidney and liver diseases.
- **Toxins**: An example includes lead.
- Specific tumors or brain infections.
- Adverse reactions to medication (Leonard, 2022).
- **Vascular disorders**: These medical conditions affect your brain's blood circulation (WedMD, 2023). Examples of vascular disorders are traumatic brain injuries that can manifest as a result of car accidents, falls, a mild knock to the head, and more.
- **Infections in the central nervous system**: These include meningitis, Human Immunodeficiency Virus, and Creutzfeldt-Jakob disease.
- **Alcohol and drug use**: Furthermore, prolonged alcohol and drug use and specific types of hydrocephalus (i.e., a gradual accumulation of water in the brain) are other examples.

Risk Factors That Cannot be Changed

- **Age**: Those at least 65 years old and older are more likely to develop dementia (Centers for Disease Control and Prevention, 2019). However, even younger people can develop dementia.
- **Family History**: If you have parents, siblings, or other family members diagnosed with dementia, that significantly increases your chances of developing dementia (Centers for Disease Control and Prevention, 2019). However, there are people who, despite their family history of dementia, do not develop it. Then, some people who do not have a family history go on to develop dementia. It is advisable to get tested to find out whether you have specific genetic mutations that can lead to the development of dementia.

Risk Factors That Can be Changed

- **Diet and exercise**: Research reveals that a lack of exercise gives rise to the development of dementia. No study acknowledges that a particular diet helps to reduce the risk of the development of dementia. Nonetheless, there is research that shows that people who have an unhealthy diet have a greater risk of developing dementia compared to those who perhaps adopt a Mediterranean diet which is rich in

nutrients found in whole grains, fruits, seafood, nuts, beans, vegetables, and seeds.
- **Excessive alcohol use**: It is common knowledge that consuming large quantities of alcohol can lead to changes in the brain. A significant number of studies have revealed that disorders related to alcohol use are significantly associated with the development of dementia, especially early-onset dementia.
- **Cardiovascular diseases**: Examples of diseases associated with the heart and blood vessels include high blood pressure, high cholesterol levels, plaque buildup in your arteries known as atherosclerosis, and having a body mass index of over 30 that can have someone be considered an obese person.
- **Depression**: Even though the risk factor of depression associated with the development of dementia is not well-researched, however, developing depression in late adulthood can lead to the development of dementia.
- **Diabetes**: Being diabetic can significantly increase one's likelihood of developing dementia, mainly if it is not in remission.
- **Smoking**: It is dangerous to one's health because it can raise one's chances of developing dementia and other diseases, such as vascular diseases.
- **Head trauma**: Experiencing a severe head injury can significantly increase a person's risk of developing Alzheimer's disease. A plethora of research shows

that people aged 50 years and older who experienced a traumatic brain injury had an increased risk of developing dementia and Alzheimer's disease. Similarly, people who have experienced more severe and many traumatic brain injuries had an increased risk of dementia and Alzheimer's disease too.
- **Sleep disturbances**: Suffering from sleep apnea and other sleep disturbances can lead to a greater risk of developing dementia.
- **Vitamin and nutritional deficiencies**: Having deficiencies in the following vitamins: D, B-6, B-12, and folate can increase your likelihood of developing dementia.
- **Medications that negatively affect memory**: Doctors recommend refraining from using over-the-counter pain relief and sleep aids that include active ingredients, such as diphenhydramine, which is commonly found in Advil PM and Aleve PM products. Also, doctors recommend refraining from using medications to treat an overactive bladder and other urinary conditions with an active ingredient known as oxybutynin sold in Ditropan XL products.

Also, try to avoid sedatives and sleeping tablets. Ask your doctor if any medications you are taking could worsen your memory.

SYMPTOMS OF DEMENTIA

Dementia symptoms present in one person may not be present in another because of the differences in the cause of the disease. However, common symptoms of dementia include:

Cognitive Changes

- **Forgetfulness or short-term memory loss**: Many people with dementia have short-term memory problems. Examples include forgetting the name of a close family member or friend, repeatedly asking the same question, forgetting old memories, and misplacing things (WebMD, 2023). Also, they can remember memories from 20 years ago as if they happened yesterday but have difficulty remembering what they ate at breakfast (Leonard, 2022).
- **Difficulty with visual and spatial abilities**: Suffering from dementia can cause difficulties in reading text, stereoscopic vision, and determining distances, color, or contrast. For example, someone with dementia can get lost while driving in a familiar neighborhood or not know how they got to a particular place. Also, they can confuse the difference between day and night (ADI, n.d.b.).
- **Problems with language; difficulty with finding the right words**: People with dementia can struggle with remembering the right words to use in

expressing themselves (Leonard, 2022) or using strange words to associate with objects they know and use every day (Centers for Disease Control and Prevention, 2019).
- **Difficulty performing familiar tasks or inability to complete tasks independently**: Someone with dementia can experience difficulty completing routine tasks that they usually perform daily or have performed for several years. Also, people living with dementia can struggle with knowing the order of what clothing items to wear first and last or the steps for making a cup of coffee (ADI, n.d.b; Leonard, 2022).
- **Problems with concentration, planning, or organizing**: Someone with dementia might struggle with making decisions, solving problems, or paying their bills on time (ADI, n.d.b).
- **Problems with reasoning and judgment**: People with dementia might struggle with wearing appropriate clothes for events, or they could put on too many layers of clothing on a hot day or wear too few clothes on a day with freezing weather (ADI, n.d.b.).

Psychological Changes

- **Personality, mood, or behavioral changes**: Everyone experiences fluctuations in their mood,

from sadness to frustration, from time to time. People with dementia can feel emotions in ways that are not normal for them and have rapid mood swings or agitation without cause for it. Also, they can show less emotion or act up in social interactions than before (ADI, n.d.b.).
- **Depression, paranoia, anxiety, or hallucinations**: Mental health problems are common for people with dementia (Leonard, 2022; WebMD, 2023).
- **Withdrawal from socializing**: People living with dementia may sometimes not feel up to cleaning the house, attending meetings, or going to social gatherings. Nonetheless, someone living with dementia can become very passive, which others will notice about them. For example, they can spend hours watching television, sleeping too much, or seemingly have lost interest in their hobbies (ADI, n.d.b.).

I [Connolly] had a close friend whose grandmother, Gertrude, had lived in an old-age home for the past year and a half (Conolly, 2016). One day she had a visitor, her son, who took some highly scented flowers called Fragrant Daphne. Her son hoped that she would have been able to remember when she grew them in her house years ago. The refreshing citrus perfume of the flowers brought nature into her room. She said, "Thank you, my sweetheart. I think I have been planting those here." A split second later, she forgets about the bunch of flowers and then becomes worried about the events she had scheduled and is confused about whether it is a Monday or Wednesday.

I had another friend whose mother-in-law, Cathy, would have visitations from my friend named Victoria and her husband. My friend's job was shopping with Cathy on Tuesdays every week. However, Cathy would find pleasure in taking *my friend* out for lunch. Cathy loved her daughter-in-law since she never had a daughter, but always wanted one. Regardless of her confused mind, she always looked forward to Tuesday, as it was Victoria's Day.

There was an incident Victoria retold to me about Cathy calling her about the daily newspaper. To her, it seemed the publishers printed the incorrect date on the newspaper. She felt disoriented by the wrong date printed on the newspaper. It was difficult for Victoria to persuade her that the date was correct and that she was mistaken. It was evident that she had trouble with reasoning and remembering what date it was when she received the newspaper.

SUMMARY

- Dementia is called a "silent thief" because it progressively removes memories from a person's mind without them knowing about it.
- *Dementia* is a broad term with many definitions from academic and non-academic sources. Simply put,

dementia is a syndrome with many underlying symptoms with several causes for the deterioration in cognitive functioning that affects a person's daily, social or occupational functioning.
- Causes of dementia vary from bodily diseases, injuries, and specific disorders to medication side effects and toxins.
- There are primarily two risk factors that cannot be changed: Age and family history. Several risk factors can be changed, such as diet and exercise, excessive alcohol use, cardiovascular disease, depression, diabetes, smoking, head trauma, sleep disturbances, vitamin and nutritional deficiencies, and medications that negatively affect memory.
- Symptoms of dementia can have cognitive and psychological changes. The mental changes include forgetfulness, difficulty with visual and spatial abilities, problems with language, performing familiar tasks, concentration, planning or organizing, reasoning, and judgment. Also, the psychological changes include personality, mood or behavioral changes, mental health disorders, such as depression, paranoia, anxiety or hallucinations, and withdrawal from socializing.
- Two anecdotes were highlighted about Jean and Cathy, suffering from dementia, and some of their symptoms, such as confusion and disorientation in time.

While dementia is among senior citizen's most discussed conditions, many misconceptions exist. For instance, when people hear of dementia, they often immediately think it is synonymous with Alzheimer's disease. However, Alzheimer's is only one type of dementia. In addition, some are unaware of the different stages of dementia. Understanding dementia's different types and stages is crucial—it will help you determine the best care for your loved one suffering from this condition.

Thus, in the next chapter, you will explore the various types of dementia and how they differ. You will also get an insight into the different stages of dementia, including the symptoms for each, so you can know what to expect as the condition progresses.

3

DISCOVERING THE MANY FACES OF DEMENTIA

According to Alzheimer's Disease International, across the globe, there are over 41 million people who have symptoms of dementia, but they have not received a formal diagnosis (Gregory & Geddes, 2021).

It is extremely crucial to receive a formal diagnosis of dementia to allow people who live with the disease to receive the treatment and support they need, which is better to receive at the beginning of the disease rather than when the symptoms are worse as the disease progresses.

An interesting piece of research from McGill University, located in Montreal, Canada, revealed that in certain countries, more than 90 percent of people living with dementia have not received a formal diagnosis of the disease (Gregory & Geddes, 2021).

There are various types of dementia, which people may not even know about because of the lack of information in their healthcare systems, too few available trained specialists, and lack of access to diagnostic tools. High-income and middle-income countries can both experience a lack of resources on one or more of these facets, making it seem like there are low dementia cases in respective countries.

TYPES OF DEMENTIA

Every type of dementia identified and well-researched in the medical field affects a particular part of the brain, especially in the early stages of the disease (Alzheimer's Society, 2021a). That is why several symptoms are different from each other that are only present in certain types of dementia and not in other types of dementia. For example, memory loss is one of the symptoms of dementia that are found in the early stages of Alzheimer's disease. However, it is rarely found in the early stages of frontotemporal dementia.

When the disease progresses from the early stages to the middle and later stages, the symptoms in different types of dementia go from being distinct in those types of dementia to being similar over time.

As the disease progresses, it will spread to other brain areas. That will cause someone with dementia to have more symptoms due to more parts of their brain not functioning normally. As this is happening, areas of the brain that have already been damaged will be significantly affected; in turn, this will cause the affected person's symptoms to worsen.

It will get to the point where many brain areas will be immensely impaired by the disease that is causing their dementia. Unfortunately, this results in significant brain changes affecting memory, thinking abilities, language, emotions, and behavior. Sometimes it can cause problems with physical movement.

Below are examples of five types of dementia that are common, such as Alzheimer's disease, and those that are less commonly known, such as mixed dementia:

Alzheimer's Disease

It is one of the most common and widely known causes of dementia worldwide. According to the Alzheimer's Association, approximately between 60 and 80 percent of dementia cases globally are a result of Alzheimer's disease (Herndon, 2022). Most people living with dementia usually get a formal diagnosis at the age of 65 or older. If people get diagnosed before age 65, it is often clinically called "early onset dementia." Specific brain changes cause Alzheimer's disease. The symptoms include (Alzheimer's Society, 2023; Gupta, 2022; Herndon, 2022):

- Memory loss that impairs daily functioning, such as remembering the fastest route to drive home and difficulty with recalling recent events.
- Confused about where they are, what day it is, or what year it is.
- Trouble with thinking and reasoning.
- Language problems.
- Difficulty with performing familiar tasks, such as washing the dishes.
- Usually lose things and cannot backtrack their steps to find them.
- Trouble with resolving issues.
- Difficulty with their speech or writing.
- Experience disorientation in time and places.
- Reduced ability to make good judgment.
- Pay less attention to taking care of their personal hygiene.
- Have personality and mood changes.
- Lost interest in socializing with friends, family, and community.

Vascular Dementia

After Alzheimer's disease, vascular dementia is the second most common type of dementia. People living with dementia, especially vascular dementia, will experience it uniquely. Generally, vascular dementia is caused by inadequate blood flow to particular regions and subregions of the brain. Symptoms, the cause, and brain areas the disease affects will vary from person to person. There are symptoms of vascular dementia that are the same as other types of dementia. These include memory loss, difficulty with thinking, language, mood, or behavioral changes. Nonetheless, symptoms of vascular dementia can present differently and even subtly or suddenly at first and then progressively worsen over time. The symptoms include (Alzheimer's Society, 2022a; Hill, 2022a; Holland, 2022):

- Difficulty making plans, good judgments, organizing, decision-making, and problem-solving.
- Memory problems that disrupt your loved one's daily life.
- Problems following step-by-step instructions, such as making a cheese-grilled sandwich with sliced tomatoes.
- Confusion or agitation.
- Trouble with performing tasks they used to do and found easy.
- Slower thinking.
- Difficulties with concentration.
- Difficulty with their speech or understanding speech, commonly known as Aphasia.
- Difficulty with physical movement as it affects a person's muscles and coordination, a health condition known as Apraxia.
- Trouble recognizing familiar people, sounds, or objects is a health condition known as Agnosia.

- Trouble with processing information while performing other tasks and recalling instructions.
- Mood and personality changes include problems with walking and falling too many times.

There are many instances where people living with vascular dementia will have difficulty staying employed, performing household duties, or maintaining social relationships. People with vascular dementia can experience neurological symptoms, such as hyperreflexia, which refers to hyperactive reflexes, difficulty with walking, running, and balance, and slight loss of feeling in their arms, legs, hands, and feet.

Some people with vascular dementia, depending on the etiology of dementia, can have further symptoms such as hallucinations, urinary problems, and depression.

Frontotemporal Dementia

Frontotemporal dementia is otherwise known as Pick's disease or frontal lobe dementia. Other names for frontotemporal dementia are Frontotemporal degeneration, Temporal dementia, Pick's complex, Frontotemporal lobar degeneration, and Frontal dementia. Frontotemporal dementia is one of the least common types of dementia. Frontotemporal dementia refers to disorders that can result in changes in emotions, behavior, thinking, and communication caused by a slow drop in nerve cells over time in the frontal or temporal lobes of the brain. The symptoms include (Alzheimer's Society, n.d.a; Heerema, 2021a; Holland, 2017):

- Changes in personality and behavior, such as making insensitive comments, decreased sense of empathy, lack of interest in activities, difficulty good personal hygiene and care, or exhibiting compulsive behavior.
- A lack of self-control out of nowhere in interpersonal and social interactions.
- Trouble with finding the right words to express themselves verbally, which can make an individual feel less confident to speak, and they can, in turn, try to speak slowly.
- Difficulty understanding speech, may affect their ability to form meaningful sentences to respond to what others are saying or affect their ability to read and write and may cause trouble with language recall.
- Physical problems with moving and controlling their limbs, hands, and feet, such as experiencing trembling sensations, muscle spasms, and difficulty balancing themselves (e.g., they may frequently fall).

Lewy Body Dementia

Lewy body dementia is a type of dementia caused by Lewy bodies, which are tiny deposits of a protein that forms in the brain. It is a medical condition that occurs when deposits form in the part of the brain called the cortex. The symptoms include (Alzheimer's Society, 2021b; Hill, 2022b; Pietrangelo, 2022):

- Trouble with clear thinking, alertness, decision-making, being attentive, or staying focused.
- Memory problems.
- Experience visual hallucinations (i.e., seeing things or hearing voices that are not there in real life, especially animals and people, even though it feels natural to them in their mind).
- Unusual sleepiness during the daytime.
- Unusual bursts of energy.
- Experience depression, agitation, and anxiety.
- Fluctuations in autonomic bodily functions, including blood pressure, body temperature, and bladder and bowel movements.
- Trouble with frequent falls.
- Periods of "blanking out" or staring.
- Trouble with physically moving their limbs, hands, and feet, as well as shaking, slowness, stooped posture, muscle stiffness, and difficulty walking.
- Experience vivid dreams whereby they act out physically, including talking, falling out of bed, walking, and kicking, commonly known as Rapid Eye Movement (REM) sleep behavior disorder.
- Trouble with maintaining a self-care routine after years of the symptoms mentioned above begins.

Mixed Dementia

Mixed dementia combines two types of dementia (Heerema, 2021b). It is usually a combination of Alzheimer's disease and vascular dementia. The symptoms of this type of dementia can progress faster or even appear earlier than the other types because the brain is impaired in more than one part, and they experience more than one difficulty.

STAGES OF DEMENTIA

Dementia comprises multiple illnesses, notably different types of physical diseases that affect the brain, such as Alzheimer's disease, vascular dementia, frontotemporal dementia, and Lewy body dementia (Alzheimer's Society, 2021a). The early stages of all the different yet similar types of dementia you have learned about in the earlier section of this chapter have one thing: Only a small area of the brain gets affected. At this point, the person affected with dementia experiences few symptoms as the parts of the brain affected by the disease only have impaired a few of their cognitive abilities. Many neurologists usually refer to these early symptoms as "mild" dementia instead of the "early" stage because they are relatively insignificant.

Every type of dementia damages a particular part of the brain in the early stage. That is the reason for the varying symptoms of the various types of dementia. For instance, memory loss is commonly experienced in the early stages of

Alzheimer's disease, but it is rarely experienced in the early stages of frontotemporal dementia.

When the disease-causing dementia progresses into the middle and later stages of the different types of dementia, its symptoms tend to become more or less the same. It becomes the case because more brain parts become affected over time.

As dementia progresses, it affects other brain areas. Thus, more symptoms are experienced by the person with dementia because more parts of the brain have difficulty functioning normally. At the same time, brain areas that have been impaired become more damaged than they already had been before, causing the person to experience worse symptoms than before the disease-causing dementia spread to other brain areas over time.

In the end, many brain areas get significantly impaired by the disease that causes dementia. Unfortunately, this causes significant changes to a person's memory, thinking, language, emotions, problem-solving, perception, behavior, and physical problems.

It is essential to learn about the stages of dementia because when you care for someone with dementia, they will need more assistance over time. At a particular stage, they will need significant support in their daily activities to stay alive. However, dementia affects people differently, so there is no way to determine how soon this will happen for your loved one and what kind of support they need (Alzheimer's Society, 2021a). Also, defining the stage helps physicians to decide on the best treatments and allows them communicate with doctors and caregivers (Dementia Care Central, 2023). The different stages of dementia guide when specific treatments, such as medicines for Alzheimer's disease, are likely to work best.

Dementia usually has three stages of progression, namely, mild (or "early stage"), moderate ("middle stage"), and severe ("late stage"). There is a more scientifically defined way to determine the specific stage of dementia the disease has progressed to by using the Global Deterioration Scale or the Reisberg Scale. These scales divide the development of dementia over time into seven clearly defined stages based on the significant amount of cognitive deterioration.

Below, these seven stages are elaborated on as follows (Alzheimer's Association, n.d.a; DailyCaring Editorial Team, n.d.a; Dayton, 2021; Dementia Care Central, 2023; Frontier Management, n.d.; Ivy Palmer Live-in Care Services, n.d.; Leonard, 2022; MacGill, 2023; WHO, 2023):

No Dementia or Preclinical Stage

- This preclinical stage will see the patient experience symptoms that range from no cognitive deterioration (stage one) to very mild cognitive deterioration (stage two) and mild cognitive deterioration (stage three).

- Research has shown that the brain goes through changes before the person with dementia experiences symptoms that are apparent to themselves and others. During this preclinical stage, dementia and its symptoms are challenging to detect.
- At this preclinical stage, the dementia patient may not need to receive care once they receive a formal diagnosis of dementia. However, they will need care as the disease progresses and their symptoms worsen.
- This preclinical stage can last between two and seven years.

Early Dementia Stage

- This early dementia stage will see the patient experience symptoms of moderate cognitive deterioration (stage four).
- At this early dementia stage, the dementia patient has received their formal diagnosis. They will start sensing that something is amiss, and usually, they notice that they are being more forgetful than usual.
- They may need little care and can live alone without being a danger to themselves and others around them. However, they may need help to develop coping strategies for their initial symptoms and secure their safety.

- This early dementia stage can last, on average, for two years.

Middle Dementia Stage

- This middle dementia stage will see the patient experience symptoms that range from moderately severe cognitive deterioration (stage five) to severe cognitive deterioration (stage six).
- Memory loss becomes more pervasive and increases. People with dementia usually experience this stage longer than the preclinical and early dementia stages.
- During this middle dementia stage, the person affected with dementia may need help to perform their daily activities, such as taking a shower, grooming, and wearing appropriate clothes. Also, it is in this stage of dementia that it becomes dangerous to leave the dementia patient alone. That means they will need supervision.
- This middle dementia stage can last, on average, for one and a half to two and a half years.

Late Dementia Stage

- This late dementia stage will see the patient experience symptoms of very severe cognitive deterioration (stage seven).

- The dementia patient will become more dependent and lose their identity. They might lose awareness of their surroundings, making it difficult to respond to and recognize their surroundings, family members, and caregivers.
- At this late dementia stage, the dementia patient will need significant care around the clock. They will be utterly dependent on their caregiver and need help and supervision 24 hours, seven days a week. They will not be able to perform any daily activities on their own.
- This late dementia stage can last, on average, for one and a half to two and a half years.

In the earlier chapters, it was mentioned that Robin Williams suffered from Lewy body dementia. His widow tells how her husband lived with this disease (Williams, 2016). Robin and Susan had unconditional love for one another. Susan supported her husband and helped him as he began to deteriorate slowly. The early indicators of Lewy body dementia that Robin experienced were extreme feelings of anxiety and fear resulting from a large amount of Lewy bodies in his amygdala. His wife wished Robin knew that he had a neurological disease that was the cause of his struggles; it was not his fault.

He was a Julliard-trained actor and had been in many movies. While filming *Night at the Museum 3*, his doctor prescribed him antipsychotic medication to manage his anxiety. However, it worsened his symptoms instead of helping them. Also, when filming for this movie, he would forget his lines, which was devastating. She tried to help him see his brilliance, but his memory loss made him insecure. Highly intelligent people generally appear to be fine when the symptoms of Lewy body dementia begin.

Robin became aware he was losing his mind. She did not know how much he was suffering and fighting for his life. As his wife, Susan felt powerless and did not know whether her husband was facing one cause of the disease or many underlying causes of his illness.

Later on in his life, he was formally diagnosed with Parkinson's disease. For a while, he tried "doing all the right things," from psychotherapy, physical therapy, exercising, and meditation to yoga to alleviate some of his symptoms, but nothing worked. His wife recalls he had these symptoms: Tremors, a slow, shuffling gait, difficulty finding the right words in conversations, insomnia, frozen stance, trouble with visuospatial abilities and basic reasoning, and confusion. These symptoms would come and go at random times.

Sadly, Robin experienced almost all of the over 40 symptoms of Lewy body dementia, except he never had hallucinations. Often, when doctors diagnose a disease, it is always the case that the disease has been progressing for quite some time.

Susan remembers the last time Robin said "Goodnight, my love" when they were about to sleep. It was the last she would see of him as her beloved passed away on Monday, August 11, 2014.

She committed herself to continuing their research to understand the science behind his condition. After performing an autopsy, doctors confirmed that he suffered from diffuse Lewy body dementia, which means nearly every part of his brain was invaded by an abnormal clumping of the protein called α-synuclein. That helped her to understand that a patient can be diagnosed with Lewy body dementia instead of Parkinson's disease and vice versa, depending on the symptoms that appear first. Her husband was clinically diagnosed with Parkinson's disease and pathologically had symptoms of diffuse Lewy body dementia.

Susan went on to serve on the Board of Directors of the American Brain Foundation.

SUMMARY

- There are over 41 million people with dementia worldwide, and more than 90 percent of them have not been formally diagnosed with the disease.
- There are four primary types of dementia, which affect different brain areas and have varying symptoms. As the disease progresses, the symptoms become more or less the same between the different types of dementia.

- The four primary types of dementia are Alzheimer's disease, vascular dementia, Lewy body dementia, and Frontotemporal dementia. The fifth type of dementia is mixed dementia, which is commonly a combination between Alzheimer's disease and vascular dementia.
- Alzheimer's trademark symptom is difficulty recalling recent events, amongst other symptoms. Vascular dementia has symptoms ranging from trouble with speaking, recognizing sights and sounds, to changes in personality and mood. Frontotemporal dementia affects movement and the ability to control your behavior in personal and social situations, amongst other symptoms. Lewy body dementia impairs executive functioning and causes visual hallucinations, problems with movement, and other symptoms.
- There are seven stages of dementia. All types of dementia start by affecting a small brain area, and then, over time, the symptoms worsen as more areas of the brain get damaged.
- Susan Williams, the wife of the late Robin Williams, shares her story of supporting her husband in his battles with his clinical diagnosis of Parkinson's disease and pathology of diffuse Lewy body dementia.

Because of the effects of dementia on one's brain, the condition significantly impacts a person's thinking, behavior, and ability to perform even the simplest tasks. Coping with the symptoms of dementia can be difficult and overwhelming, not just for the person suffering from it, but for their loved ones as well.

In the next chapter, you will explore the effects of dementia on one's emotions, behaviors, and relationships.

4

IDENTIFYING THE IMPACT OF DEMENTIA

Over 11 million Americans care for their loved ones with Alzheimer's or other types of dementia without compensation (Alzheimer's Association, 2023b). In 2021, it was estimated that these caregivers were estimated to have spent over 16 billion hours taking care of their loved ones with dementia, which amounted to a hefty $272 billion. Since women are the nurturers in society, they make up two-thirds of the caregivers. To further support this point, more than one-third of caregivers of people with dementia are daughters. It is estimated that 66 percent of caregivers live with their loved ones with dementia in the community. Nearly one-third of these caregivers take care not only of their loved one with dementia, which is most likely to be one of their parents or both but also if they are parents themselves, they will care for their child or children. It is commendable how caregivers give so much of themselves to care for their loved ones with dementia. However, it can be strenuous and overwhelming for caregivers in many areas of their lives to take care of loved ones with dementia. Twice as many caregivers of people with dementia experience significant emotional, financial, and physical struggles compared to caregivers who do not live with dementia.

EFFECTS OF DEMENTIA ON THE PERSON WITH THE CONDITION

It is always best to gain an understanding of a condition that someone you love is living with to help support them with it in the best way possible (Alzheimer's Society, 2022b). Also, it builds compassion and empathy toward people who may be different, which helps to foster understanding and makes your loved one living with a condition feel seen. It can be challenging to witness your loved one experience changes in personality, emotions, behavior, and even physical, beyond your and their control. It is very helpful when caregivers, friends, and family can assist the person with the condition receive the help they need to maintain a good quality of life despite their condition.

Emotional Effects

When someone has received a formal diagnosis of dementia, they are most likely to feel a range of emotions from anger, grief, and denial to terror and shock (Better Health, 2014b).

They could experience depression and anxiety from receiving the confirmation of their diagnosis. They may rarely feel comforted by the confirmation of their diagnosis, but that could be possible for people who are self-aware and have noticed strange changes within themselves. If your loved one struggles to manage their emotions, it could be due to being scared about what will happen to them and those around them. How will their future be living with this condition? How will they control or even notice moments of confusion and forgetfulness? Will their loved ones be safe around them? These could be some of the questions they may be initially asking themselves, which talking to a counselor or finding a support group could help to acknowledge their feelings and concerns.

Effects on Self-Esteem

People with dementia may feel insecure and less confident in themselves and performing everyday tasks. Suppose word gets out about their diagnosis to the community and extended family members. In that case, they may feel stigmatized and socially isolated because others may treat them differently due to their condition, especially those who may not care about them as much. Changes to their physical health, financial situation, employment, social status, friendships, and family relationships that they value can negatively affect their self-esteem. Caregivers can use techniques and approaches to reduce the impact of these changes on their self-esteem and help their loved one keep a normal lifestyle and routine for as long as possible (Alzheimer's Society, 2022b).

Mental and Behavioral Effects

People living with dementia experience difficulties with their memory and thinking abilities (Alzheimer's Society, 2022b). That can negatively affect their self-esteem and acceptance and trust in themselves, social status and relationships, and the ability to engage in their hobbies and use everyday life skills, such as cooking, laundry, driving, and hair styling.

As the disease gradually worsens, people living with dementia may begin to behave in ways that are difficult to understand and socially inappropriate for themselves and others around them. For instance, they can become restless or irritated, scream out of nowhere, become paranoid and suspect others are out to get them, follow people around, and ask the same question repeatedly.

Communicating

Most people living with dementia typically experience difficulties with their speech and understanding and responding to others communicating with them (Alzheimer's Society, 2022b). For example, as mentioned in the previous chapter, they can experience trouble finding the right words to express themselves or concentrating enough to follow a conversation. Beyond these factors, several other factors can affect communication, such as pain, shame, side effects of certain medications, other mental and medical conditions, and sensory impairments.

Nonetheless, the person living with dementia will still possess some of their abilities even though they may be diminished in nature. They will still be able to have an emotional connection to those around them and their environment, even when the condition gets to its late stages.

EFFECTS OF DEMENTIA ON A PERSON'S LOVED ONES OR CAREGIVERS

People who have their loved ones diagnosed with dementia have a story of that moment they heard of the news (Britton, n.d.). It is more common for caregivers to have felt either one or more of these emotions, such as relief of knowing what is wrong, involuntary tearfulness with a close family member after hearing the news in the car, or even unemotional as you choose to get on with life, anger at what is happening to your loved one, complete denial as you may have believed that the doctor is wrong, and any other emotion that one can have upon confirmation of a diagnosis.

Reasons for Emotional Impact

Generally, caregivers who are the family members of the person diagnosed with dementia have too much on their plates (DementiaUK, 2020). They will also need to take on different responsibilities in their role as a caregiver for their loved ones with dementia. If the person with dementia is a family member, they will become the center of attention because everyone will want to ensure their needs are met. That can cause other family members, such as children and spouses (if they have a family of their own), to feel neglected and resentful because they are not getting quality time and meeting their needs, even though this may not be intentional from the caregiver's perspective. They may be the one who is responsible for everyday tasks, such as cooking, chores, and helping the children with their homework, and that can feel like a burden when you need to take care of someone else. Unfortunately, some caregivers can withdraw from social gatherings with friends and family, or if they are married, their spouse could file for a divorce.

Emotional Impact on Loved Ones

Many people affected by the diagnosis of dementia of a loved one, whether a friend or a relative, can experience a myriad of emotional responses to the confirmation of it that can range from denial, fear, guilt, anger, and frustration to grief and loss, which is distressful to themselves and those around them.

Denial

It is rare to find people who want to confront the reality of either themselves or their loved one with a terminal health condition (Britton, n.d.). Being in denial is a way to cushion oneself from what is happening. With time, they become accepting of the condition and will be able to seek information about the condition to educate themselves on living with this condition.

Fear

Fear is an emotional response that results from feeling helpless and powerless. Fear is associated with dementia in different ways, such as the fear of having people notice those initial symptoms (i.e., being concerned with what people will say). They can also experience the fear of wondering what the future will hold, and as the disease progresses, the fear of what might happen next to them can become apparent. Some things that can help eliminate fear are putting together a detailed and well-researched early plan for care and seeking support from organizations. Also, thinking about an advanced care plan and Power of Attorney are great strategies to manage fear in this context.

Guilt

Loved ones with a family member living with dementia can experience guilt associated with the decisions they need to make about the care of their loved ones. Many families feel guilty if doctors tell them they must take their family member to a care facility, especially if they do not have the means to care for their loved one.

Grief and Loss

Grief is an emotional response to loss (Alzheimer's Society of Canada, n.d.). In the context of a loved one diagnosed with dementia, family members are faced with the loss of the person their loved one used to be, and their relationship with them can be affected. People caring for their spouse can experience grief at the loss of the future they could have shared with their partner.

Anger and Frustration

It is normal to feel angry at everyone and everything. For example, a caregiver can be angry at their situation of needing to care for someone with dementia. If there are people who are meant to be helping but are not doing that, it can cause anger and frustration. Also, it is normal to feel angry and frustrated at the challenging behaviors of a person with dementia and support services and organizations.

EFFECTS OF DEMENTIA ON A PERSON'S RELATIONSHIP WITH LOVED ONES

Different people will react differently to a loved one diagnosed with dementia. Some might be helpful, whereas others will want to distance themselves from the person with dementia and the family. That happens because they often feel they cannot cope with seeing their loved one deteriorate before their eyes. Conversely, some people will come to develop a close relationship with their loved one with dementia and work with them to solve their problems. Interestingly, these people will get to learn about strengths they never knew they had before.

Impact on Couples or Intimacy

When a partner or spouse is diagnosed with dementia, it is normal not to know how to act or react. Couples come a long way with their partner and have strong emotional ties to them, which can affect how they act and react to their partner diagnosed with dementia. Here are some ideas for dealing with a partner with dementia:

- Do not allow the diagnosis to rule over your lives together. Still, make plans to travel the world, go on date nights, and do fun activities.
- Seek professional couples counseling to help with getting through this.
- Plan ahead for medical and financial concerns. Arrange meetings with an attorney, a financial advisor, or family members to see how best to plan for your wishes to be legally written and known by family members.

Impact on Children

Children often do not get detailed explanations of the disease that may affect at least one of their parents or a close relative. Also, children may not receive the same attention as they may have been accustomed to when much of the focus and attention of the family goes to the person with dementia.

Children can react differently when they hear that a parent or someone else in the family has dementia. Younger children may fear that they will be diagnosed with the condition or that they are responsible for their family members getting the disease. On the other hand, teenagers could feel resentful if assigned more responsibilities or embarrassed when their loved one starts to act strangely in front of other people. Young adults, possibly in their college years, may not want to leave home.

Children often need reassurance, straightforwardness about the disease, and support to manage their emotions. So, setting up a meeting with the doctor, a school counselor, and teachers to notify them of what is going on in their lives and encouraging them to attend support groups for their age group can be helpful for children.

Impact on Other Family Members and Friends

Other family members and friends may not be accepting of the condition. People with dementia can feel resentful if they lack support from other family members who cannot help them for whatever reason. Friends, on the other hand, may choose never to speak to or spend time with the person with dementia because they do not know what to say to them, or they could be worried about the person's emotions and behaviors. Alternatively, they can choose to be there for them in whatever way their friend needs them during a time they need them the most.

Precious shares a story of caring for a loved one with dementia (Nehring, 2016). Precious was married to John for 47 years when she was told that her husband had been diagnosed with the early onset of Alzheimer's disease. A few things helped their partnership to face the struggles they experienced, such as accepting the confirmation of the diagnosis, loving and respecting each other, maintaining their faith in God, putting each other's needs above their own, never giving up, laughing a lot and hoping for advances in scientific and medical research.

One of the early symptoms of the disease that Precious noticed was that John began to not stay on top of things that he usually would take care of, such as paying the electricity and water bill on time. At first, when such things he used to do were declining, she immediately was in denial. However, later on, they went on to seek help from an organization that supports people with Alzheimer's.

For John, he knew something was wrong with him but could not put his finger on it. The first time he noticed something might be wrong was when he took 20 minutes to deposit money into his bank account, which was unusual for him as he would do it very quickly before.

After noticing his problems with everyday tasks, Precious took John to get help. He was initially diagnosed with Mild Cognitive Impairment and later correctly diagnosed with Alzheimer's disease.

The biggest challenge to their relationship was the role reversal for Precious because she now had to take on John's responsibilities in their relationship and household, such as taking care of the finances, driving, and other responsibilities. Whereas John's biggest challenge was not being able to care for his wife as he used to and forgetting the everyday details; for example, he had a problem with forgetting to eat even though Precious put food on the table for him.

Writing everything down from appointments to reminders, doing weekly fun activities, and joining a support group for the spouse with a newly diagnosed partner are some of the strategies that helped Precious and John as a couple to manage the changes that come with the disease and to maintain a good quality life.

SUMMARY

- Over 11 million Americans care for people with Alzheimer's and other related dementia without compensation. Usually, these caregivers are primarily women and live with a person with dementia. They also suffer from significant emotional, financial, and physical struggles due to their care responsibilities.
- Dementia can affect the person with the condition emotionally, as they can experience a range of emotions from grief, anger, and denial. They can also

experience a loss in their self-esteem and confidence, social status and relationships, and day-to-day life skills. They can also experience behavioral changes, such as becoming restless or irritated, suspicious of others, and repeatedly asking the same question, which can be distressing to the person with dementia and those around them. Communicating can be difficult for people living with dementia.
- Dementia on a person's loved ones or caregivers can affect them emotionally because they must take on more responsibilities and potentially neglect their children and spouse. They could feel burdened and end up withdrawing from social gatherings and family activities, and if they are married, their partner could divorce them.
- Loved ones with a family member or friend with dementia can be in denial initially and, with time, can accept the diagnosis. They can also fear people noticing their symptoms, what the future will hold, and what will happen to them. The decisions they need to make about taking care of their loved one with dementia can cause them to feel guilty, especially if they need to let a care facility take care of their loved one. Also, loved ones can feel grief and loss of the person their loved one was before the disease and the relationship they had with them. They could feel angry and frustrated with everything and everyone involved with the disease, such as

needing to take care of the person with dementia, the person's challenging behavior, and support services.
- The impact of dementia on couples can affect how the spouse who finds out their partner is diagnosed with dementia may not know how to react or act. Children can feel neglected and resentful if they must take on different responsibilities, and older children may not want to leave home. Other family members and friends may not accept the condition and decide not to help. Alternatively, they can accept the condition and choose to be there at this most challenging time for their family member or friend affected with dementia.
- Precious tells the story of living with her husband, John, of over 47 years, who was diagnosed with Alzheimer's.

To say that dementia is difficult for both the patient and their loved ones is an understatement. As discussed in this chapter, the condition can push the patient and their loved ones to a breaking point. However, there are plenty of ways to help ease the negative impact of dementia and manage its symptoms to preserve relationships.

In the next chapter, you will explore different ways to communicate properly with a person suffering from dementia.

5

BREAKING DOWN BARRIERS

In an interview on ITV Good Morning Britain, John Barnes, a former professional football player from the United Kingdom, tells the story about how his family experienced struggles when they found out his aunt was formally diagnosed with dementia (Buntajova, 2022). He recounts how the confirmation of his aunt's diagnosis was out of the blue. His aunt was a talented dancer, enjoyed playing squash, and after 18 months from the time of the interview, she was diagnosed with dementia. Her life and the family's lives changed forever after knowing her diagnosis. He advocated that families with dementia patients need to receive support, too, not only the affected person, because families often experience too many struggles to bear on their own.

COMMUNICATION AND DEMENTIA: A REVIEW

Communication with a dementia patient is important. Effective communication is a crucial aspect of living well upon confirmation of a diagnosis of dementia. It is helpful for people living with dementia to maintain a sense of self, their social and family relationships, and good quality of life.

As dementia gets progressively worse, the person affected can expect their ability to communicate to gradually diminish in the following ways (Alzheimer's Association, n.d.b; Mayo Clinic, 2021):

- Trouble with finding the right words in conversation.
- Substituting words.
- Repeated usage of familiar words, repeating stories or questions.
- Mixing ideas, sentences, or unrelated phrases.
- Giving descriptions of familiar objects instead of naming them.
- Quickly forgetting what they wanted to say.
- Trouble with organizing words coherently and logically.
- Reverting to speaking in their mother tongue or a native language.
- Becoming a woman or a man of few words.
- Relying more on gestures to get through conversations than speaking.

Communication with someone living with dementia requires patience, compassion, and good listening skills. Below are strategies that can help you and your loved one living with dementia to understand one another better:

Communicating in the Early Stage

Dementia in the early stage is referred to as moderate cognitive deterioration, as discussed in an earlier chapter. People diagnosed with early-onset dementia can engage in meaningful conversations and social interactions. Nonetheless, they may repeat stories or questions, have trouble finding the right words to express themselves, and feel overwhelmed by plenty of stimulation. Below are some strategies that can help with communicating with someone in the early stage of dementia:

- Refrain from assuming anything concerning a person's ability to communicate as a result of knowing about their dementia diagnosis. Each person is affected differently.
- Include the person with dementia in conversations.
- Do not speak to the caregiver of the person affected by the disease when you can directly address them.
- Patiently listen to him, or her express their views, feelings, or needs.
- Take time to listen for their response rather than interrupting them.

- Ask what they are comfortable doing and what they may need your assistance with rather than assuming.
- Find out their communication preference, whether face-to-face, via email, online, or via phone calls.
- Have a laugh or two because humor always lightens the mood and helps to build a connection.
- Do not be afraid to offer your candor, friendship, encouragement, and support to the person because it might be what they were looking for too.

Communicating in the Middle Stage

Dementia in the middle stage is referred to as moderately severe cognitive deterioration, as discussed in an earlier chapter, because it can last several years. As the disease progressively worsens, the person affected will have significant trouble communicating and need more care. Below are some strategies that can help with communicating with someone in the middle stage of dementia:

- Have a conversation with the person in a quiet space with no distractions.
- Speak slowly because it makes communication easier.
- Keep eye contact, as it shows you are paying attention to what they say.
- Allow the person enough time to respond to what you are saying.

- Offer reassurance to encourage the person to continue saying what they are thinking.
- Do not ask multiple questions at a time.
- Ask simple questions that garner "yes" or "no" answers. For instance, you could ask them, "Do you want a cup of tea?" instead of "What do you feel like drinking?"
- Try to avoid over-analyzing or correcting what the person said. Rather, listen to understand what the person is saying and ask questions for clarification.
- Do not argue with the person if they say something you disagree with at your core. Instead, let it slide.
- Give step-by-step instructions if you want the person to perform any task.
- Offer visual cues when you want the person to participate in a task.
- Have written notes on standby just in case they are confused by the spoken words.

Communicating in the Late Stage

Dementia in the late stage is often referred to as severe cognitive deterioration, as discussed in an earlier chapter, and may last between several weeks to years. As the person experiences the late stage of dementia, they may use more non-verbal communication, such as facial expressions or vocal sound effects. At this late stage, the person needs care 24 hours and seven days a week. Below are some strategies that can help with communicating with someone in the late stage of dementia:

- Directly approach the person in front of their face so that they know whom they are talking to immediately.
- Encourage the person to use non-verbal gestures if you do not understand what the person is trying to get across to you.
- You can use physical touch, visual cues, vocal sound effects, smells, and tastes to communicate with the person.
- Think about the emotions behind the words you use because sometimes the emotions behind what we say can be more important than what you have said.
- Respect the person's dignity and speak to the person instead of speaking down to them or if they are not present in the room.
- If you do not know what to say, that is OK. Sometimes your being there and friendship are more important than spoken words.

VERBAL COMMUNICATION

There are many things to consider to boost the confidence of someone with dementia to start a conversation or even keep engaging with you or others in a social context. Some things to consider are the following (Clayton, 2017; Mayo Clinic, 2021; National Health System [NHS], 2023):

- Ensure you are in a setting that can facilitate good communication. For example, it would be ideal to be in a calm environment with natural lighting, and any distractions, such as the radio or the television, should be switched off.
- Be flexible and adaptable when the person is having difficulties.
- Ensure the other person's needs are met, such as ensuring they are not thirsty, hungry, or sitting uncomfortably.
- Be intentional about the time you spend with them. Spending quality time with them will make it worthwhile for both of you.

When communicating with them, you can use these techniques:

- Do not use jargon, long and complex words, and sentences that are difficult to understand.
- Try to get them to focus on you before speaking.
- Try to speak to the person conversationally rather than asking one question after the other as if they are being interviewed for a job.
- In conversations with others, ensure to include the person to make them feel valued, less isolated, and

seen.
- Now, this depends on the person; if they find long conversations tiresome, shorter conversations would be better to keep their attention.
- Use a light-hearted tone of voice while speaking to be warm and welcoming toward them.

Listening is a skill necessary for communicating with and responding to someone with dementia. Below are some strategies to use to sharpen those listening skills:

- Focus on and pay attention to what they are saying and give verbal and non-verbal encouragement.
- If you have difficulty understanding what they have said to you, ask them to say what they said again. If it is still difficult to comprehend what they are saying, rephrase what they just said and check with them if you understood what they meant to say.
- If they have trouble finding the right words or finishing sentences, kindly ask them to rephrase what they want to say differently. Pay attention and listen out for the nuances.

NON-VERBAL COMMUNICATION

Communication is more than just a verbal exchange of views, ideas, feelings, and opinions. There are other ways to convey meaning, such as gestures, body language, and facial expressions. It is usual for someone with dementia to rely on body language and physical gestures when they are struggling with their speech. Also, both of you can read and interpret each other's gestures, body language, and facial expressions. Below are some strategies to make them feel comfortable and encouraged to use non-verbal communication (DailyCaring Editorial Team, n.d.b; Mayo Clinic, 2021; NHS, 2023):

- Use physical gestures to communicate that you want to hear what the person with dementia has to say. For example, you could shake their hands, hold or pat their hand, put your arm around them, hug them, or gently rub their shoulder to reassure them. Also, check with them if they are comfortable with physical touch. You can do this by watching their body language and listening to what they say, whether they express that they are comfortable or not with your physical gestures.
- Try to have a reasonable, respectful distance from the person or stand next to them to have a conversation with them that can feel intimate.
- Ensure your gestures, body language, and facial expressions match what you are saying to avoid confusion.
- Use a positive and friendly tone of voice.
- Have a smile or a happy demeanor to make communication easier.

- If you are tall, ensure that your face is positioned at or below their eye level to make them feel like they are in control of the situation.
- Always try to maintain eye contact as best as you can.
- Project a warm and calm attitude to help the person with dementia communicate more easily.
- Visual prompts can be helpful.
- Be open to surprises. For example, the person could draw or sing what they want to express.
- Try to look out for signs of frustration, anger, or discomfort so that you can adjust your physical contact, body language, facial expressions, and responses to calm or soothe them, where possible.

OTHER TIPS

Beyond the tips already shared for verbal and non-verbal communication, there are other things you could consider to improve communication with someone with dementia, such as (Mayo Clinic, 2021; Being Patient, n.d.):

- Take a break if you feel frustrated or angry.
- Offer at least two choices when you initially ask the person something they might not agree to; for example, if the person is reluctant to go shopping, you might say, "Would you like to go shopping before or after lunch?"

- You can use technology to communicate and care for your loved one. For example, you could use tablets and smartphones with assistive technology, such as Google Home, cameras, and security systems, which can benefit the caregiver more than the person with dementia as they may not be able to use the technology at any stage of dementia.
- Do not shy away from being tearful or laughing if you feel like that at the moment.
- Use the person's name as much as possible to reassure them that "Everything is all right," especially during difficult moments.

WHAT NOT TO DO

There will be certain things that one should NOT do when caring for someone living with dementia, but also when communicating with them. Below are some things to be mindful of not doing when communicating with someone with dementia (Clayton, 2017; London, 2020):

- Generally, refrain from arguing with the person. For example, if their hallucinations and delusions frustrate you, leave the room instead of arguing with them.
- Do not order them around. If there is something you want done, do it yourself.

- Instead of telling the person what they cannot do, tell them what they can do because that will result in a productive moment for both of you.
- Even though a person with dementia may not understand spoken words, they may pick up the tone of your voice. So, please do not use a condescending tone while speaking to them.
- Someone living with dementia suffers from memory loss, amongst other symptoms they may have, so it is inconsiderate to ask many questions that will need them to rely on good memory recall.
- If you are going to talk about someone or people who are not in the room with the person with dementia, do not do it as if they are not in the room with you.
- Dementia and anger can go hand in hand for the patient and caregiver, so do not yell or raise your voice while speaking to them. The conversation can quickly escalate from a reasonably calm situation into a violent one.
- If you notice they struggle to find the right words to express themselves, give them time to try recalling a word.
- Do not dismiss their mood changes, such as looking sad or having a challenging day. Instead, let them know you see that.

SUMMARY

- John Barnes, a former professional football player from the United Kingdom, tells the story of confirming his aunt's diagnosis. He said it was sudden and advocates for families with dementia patients to receive support.
- Communication with someone with dementia is essential and can be difficult. Someone with dementia can have communication problems that range from difficulty finding their words to relying on physical touch, gestures, facial expressions, and body language more than speaking.
- There are many things to consider when communicating with someone with dementia, such as using a quiet space with minimal distractions and spending enough time with them.
- Tips were shared for verbally communicating with a person with dementia in the early, middle, and late stages of the disease.
- Strategies for non-verbal communication were shared to help you get your message across to someone with dementia through body language, physical contact, and facial expressions. The difference between verbal and non-verbal communication lies in reading the person's reaction with dementia. With verbal communication, it is essential to pay more attention to the tone and

attitude you are projecting, whereas, with non-verbal communication, it is vital to pay more attention to the physical and visual perceptions of what you are communicating with your body language, gestures, and facial expressions.

- Other tips range from taking breaks, offering at least two choices if the person is reluctant to a request, using technology to assist with communication with someone with dementia, not shying away from crying or laughing, and using their name as often as possible.
- There are many things to consider NOT doing, such as not arguing, ordering the person around, telling them what they cannot do, using a condescending tone of voice, yelling or raising your voice, dismissing their feelings, asking many questions, not giving them time to recall words to express themselves and talking about other people as if they are not there.

As mentioned, one of the changes to expect with someone suffering from dementia is difficulty finding the right words, which can be attributed to memory loss. More than communication, memory loss can also severely affect other life aspects of a person with dementia and their loved ones.

In the next chapter, you will learn simple and practical tips to help a loved one with dementia cope with memory problems.

6

DEALING WITH A FADING MEMORY

There are many interesting facts about memory. Our brains can store large amounts of information. Some experts say that our brains can store up to 2.5 petabytes of data (Greenwald, 2018). In other words, our brains can store the equivalent of 3 million hours of television programs or about the same capacity of 4,000 256 gigabytes storage on iPhones.

When the brain forgets, it is similar to walking through a doorway. When you store or retrieve information, there is a doorway that acts as an event boundary to structure how the contents are stored in long-term memory. There is a Guinness World Record for memory. Nischal Narayanam, at the tender age of 10, was awarded his first Guinness World Record for memorizing the most unfamiliar objects. He memorized a resounding 225 unfamiliar objects in a little over 12 minutes. National Geographic also recognized him as one of the seven brightest minds in the world.

Left-handed people are said to have very vivid memories in their minds. That is the case because the corpus callosum is larger in lefties, which brings together the brain's hemispheres that help to make the visuals of memories more vivid in the mind. Did you know that watching television can affect the brain? A study published in Brain and Cognition revealed that every hour a person between the ages of 40 and 59 sits in front of the television to watch programs or shows increases their risk of developing Alzheimer's disease by 1.3 percent.

DEMENTIA AND MEMORY LOSS: A REVIEW

As mentioned in an earlier chapter, dementia results from brain damage that affects certain brain areas. Thus, specific cognitive abilities get affected, such as memory (Alzheimer's Association, n.d.c). A person with dementia can experience trouble with their memory in many ways, such as difficulty creating new memories, taking longer than usual to recall information, and being unable to recall information.

In the earlier stages of dementia, the symptoms of dementia can be mild with regard to memory loss and confusion. It can be frustrating for the person experiencing these symptoms to notice the changes happening, which they have no control over, such as trouble remembering recent events, confidently making decisions, or processing what others have said.

In the later stages of dementia, memory loss, amongst other symptoms, can become significantly severe. Sadly, the person may not identify their family members, even forget relationships, call relatives by other names that are not their own, feel confused by the physical location of their home, or experience disorientation with time. They may even forget the purpose of familiar items that they use daily, such as pen and paper or a knife and fork. Caregivers and family members can find these changes painful and saddening.

HOW TO HELP YOUR LOVED ONE COPE WITH MEMORY LOSS

It is always helpful to have different strategies to tackle the challenges that may arise for your loved one with dementia and yourself when their memory begins to deteriorate. Below are some practical tips and advice to cope with memory loss as a caregiver (Alzheimer's Association, n.d.c.; Alzheimer's Society, 2021c):

- **Remain calm and patient**: If your loved one with dementia calls you by another name or they do not recognize you, that can be hurtful. However, do not let them know that it hurts you.
- **Respond with a simple explanation**: Refrain from causing the person confusion with lengthy

explanations or statements. Instead, give them a simple response that provides clarity.

- **Use visual prompts and other reminders**: Show them visual prompts and other items that can trigger the person's memory of significant relationships and places.
- **Ask few or no questions**: Asking fewer questions can help the person with dementia feel less intimidated by answering questions that do not require them to remember information.
- **Write down important pieces of information**: Writing down important pieces of information is very helpful for people with dementia because it facilitates their independence and keeping up with appointments, birthdays, reminders, and other events. Conversely, they will not forget important things even though their memories will fade away over time.
- **Travel to the place and time the person is in their mind**: If you find your loved one with dementia believes they are living in a different time or place than reality, put yourself in that particular time and place in their mind. Then, slowly engage in a conversation with them to understand their current reality and bring them to safety if they may have put themselves in a hazardous zone.
- **Make suggestions to correct their thinking**: If you notice they are confusing certain objects for others

or do not recognize family members or call them by different names, then refrain from giving them long explanations in an attempt to correct them. It will not work because they may need help understanding your long explanations. So, it is better to suggest corrections. For example, if they confuse a knife for a spoon, you could say, "I thought it was a knife." Another example is if they do not recognize their grandson, you can say, "I think he is your grandson, Cody."

- **Try not to take anything the person says too personally**: All dementia-related diseases cause the affected person to forget, feel confused, and disoriented, amongst other symptoms. So, show them your continued support and understanding despite their forgetfulness, strange behavior, and so forth because they appreciate your caring for them during this time.
- **Try to find someone or a group of trusted individuals to confide in about your experience and ask for support**: Try finding a support group, whether online or face-to-face, to share your experience with other people who may be going through the same situation as you. It will help to hear what strategies other people are using to respond to their loved ones and what works for them could work for you too. It will also help with supporting your mental wellness to have an outlet to

acknowledge your feelings and thoughts about being a caregiver.

- **Utilize memory aids and tools, such as**:

- **Post-It notes**: You can place post-it notes anywhere in your house to serve as a reminder to do a once-off task. For instance, you could place one post-it note on the refrigerator to remind you to take out the lunch you prepared for your loved one at least two hours before they need to leave the house to go to an afternoon appointment. Also, you could place another post-it note on the corridor leading to the laundry room to remind yourself to do their laundry and yours for the week.

Once you have done the task, it is vital to throw away the post-it note to ensure that you do not do the same task twice because you have accidentally reminded yourself to do a task you have already completed. Also, this will help to keep the house neat.

Once you have done the task, it is vital to throw away the post-it note to ensure that you do not do the same task twice because you have accidentally reminded yourself to do a task you have already completed. Also, this will help to keep the house neat.

- **Permanent reminders**: You can create permanent reminders, for instance, a laminated A4 sheet with reminders of important things you need to do daily written in bold letters. For example, you could place one permanent sign on the front door to remind you to take the house and car keys, handbag, wallet, or shopping list before you leave the house. Also, you could have another permanent sign near the kitchen sink to remind you to wash your hands before cooking. You could also keep another permanent sign by the bin to remind you to take it out on the day of collection.
- **Alarm clock**: Setting different alarm clocks for different tasks can be helpful. You can use a watch with an alarm or an oven timer to help remind you of things you need to remember, such as leaving the house on time for an appointment or when you leave muffins cooking in the oven and you need to check on them within 15 minutes.

Also, it is helpful to write down the reason for setting each alarm so that you do not have to wonder why it is going off in the first place. Try to keep this written reminder in a place where you are likely to walk past or quickly notice, such as a whiteboard, computer, calendar, smartphone, or diary.

- **Shopping lists**: Make a list before you leave the house to go shopping. While shopping, mark things off as you put them in your shopping basket. If you do your shopping at a particular shop regularly, then you can create a shopping list for that shop only. A friend or a family member can use these shopping lists if you need help shopping.

You can keep a list of things that have run out at home to help keep track of what you need to buy from the shops.

If you prefer to avoid writing things down, you could tear off a particular piece of the packaging of items as they run out at home. Alternatively, you could use a voice recorder app to track what you need from the shops.

- **Contact numbers**: Create a list of important and emergency contact numbers. For example:
- doctor
- community nurse
- community mental health services
- adult social care services
- care facility
- pharmacy
- dentist
- eye care specialist
- occupational therapist

- dementia adviser
- utility company
- police
- friends, family members, and neighbors
- useful community organizations

Keep this list in a suitable place, such as next to the telephone, or store them in your smartphone to easily access any services and professionals you may need to call for an emergency.

If it is available in your home country, try to find a phone that allows you to program it with all the numbers you commonly use. Then, you only need to press one digit or a button with a picture next to it to make that important call.

- **Try different medications**: Whenever your loved one that you are caring for is about to start a newly prescribed medication, it is vital to ensure their physician and pharmacist are aware of all the current medications, supplements, or other medical products they are using, as well as over-the-counter and alternative medications. It is crucial never to have specific medications interact with each other, or else it can cause serious side effects. If everything is cleared with the doctor, below are two medications that your loved one with dementia could explore to cope with their memory loss (Alzheimer's Association, n.d.d.):

- **Cholinesterase inhibitors**: These are prescribed medications that treat symptoms that pertain to memory, thinking, language, judgment, and other cognitive functions. It prevents the breakdown of acetylcholine, a chemical messenger that controls the brain centers for memory and learning.
- **Glutamate regulators**: These are prescribed medications that improve memory, awareness, logical thinking, language, and the ability to perform tasks. This medication functions by controlling the activity of glutamate, a chemical messenger that helps the brain manage data.

BRAIN EXERCISES

Medical research has proven that when people across different age groups regularly challenge their minds, their cognitive functioning is less likely to deteriorate. People who keep their minds active when they reach late adulthood can experience a shorter period of living in a state of cognitive deterioration, even if diagnosed with dementia. The science and medical fields recommend that people engage in the following activities to keep their minds active (Dementia Australia, 2016; Stuart, 2022):

- Learn something new and exciting, such as a foreign language or knitting a scarf.
- Challenging your children or grandchildren to a game of chess or any other board game. Alternatively, you can get together with friends to play a game of cards once every week. You can switch things up by trying new games. These social interactions are also great for your brain.
- Working on any kind of puzzle, such as crossword, Sudoku, and brainteasers, to name a few.
- Playing online memory games or fun video games.
- Joining local adult education classes.
- Taking up reading and writing.
- Engaging in leisure activities, such as listening to community radio stations, picking a new sport, hobby, gardening, dancing, and other fun and relaxing activities.

Crystal has been married to her husband, Cory, for 21 years and shares the story of coping with dementia in their marriage (OurParents Staff, 2023). During their marriage, Cory began to experience memory problems that changed him forever. In 2008, Cory was initially formally diagnosed with dementia and, later on, was diagnosed with Alzheimer's disease.

Crystal recalls Cory being fully present in their lives and mindful, and then one day, it was like he was not there anymore. When the doctor confirmed his diagnosis, Crystal was in denial and tearful.

As time passed and she began to accept the diagnosis and the changes happening to her husband gradually, she took steps to manage the extra responsibilities and the negative impact on her physical and mental health.

Crystal knew she would need ongoing support, which meant relying on family members, friends, professionals, or anyone willing to help. She received support from a nurse and social worker who would regularly visit their home, as well as an occupational therapist and church leader; friends and family would help her around the house and provide companionship by discussing what was going on in their lives.

To manage the stress of caregiving and the toll it took on her physical and mental health, she would prioritize taking care of her health and happiness by asking family members to stop by their home at least twice a week so that she could go to the salon to get her hair and nails done, go to medical appointments, run errands and do something she enjoys, such as buying clothes for her grandchildren.

SUMMARY

- There are many unique facts about memory, such as our brains can store up to 2.5 petabytes of information, the equivalent of 3 million hours of watching television shows; the brain can easily forget; a ten-year-old holds a Guinness World Record for memorizing 225 unfamiliar objects in little over 12 minutes, left-handed people have larger corpus callosum which makes memories more vivid in their minds. Every hour of watching television increases the risk of developing Alzheimer's disease for people between the ages of 40 and 59.

- People diagnosed with dementia can experience memory loss in different ways, such as creating new memories, retrieving information that can take longer, or not being able to retrieve anything. In the earlier stages, memory loss is mild and gets worse as the disease reaches later stages.
- There are several strategies to help your loved one with their memory loss that ranges from staying calm and patient, writing essential pieces of information down, making suggestions to correct them, finding someone or a group of trusted individuals to share your experience and ask for support, to using memory aids and tools, and trying different medications.
- Engaging in brain exercises helps to keep the mind active and reduces the time one would spend in a state of cognitive deterioration, even if one may have dementia. Many activities are recommended to keep the mind active, such as learning something new and exciting, playing board games, online memory

games, or video games, working on puzzles, joining an adult education class, reading and writing, and engaging in leisure activities.
- Crystal shares the story of coping with memory loss because of her husband's dementia.

Dealing with your loved one's memory loss due to dementia can be highly challenging, especially in the later stages of the condition. However, empowering yourself by learning what to expect and applying simple strategies can help you and your loved one cope. It is also the case for another impact of dementia—behavior changes.

In the next chapter, you will explore how to survive the struggles associated with your loved ones' changing behaviors due to dementia.

7

RESPONDING TO TROUBLING BEHAVIOR

Human behavior is compelling because of its complexities. A study on human behavior conducted in 2016 revealed that 90 percent of the human populace could be categorically classified into four basic personality types, such as Optimistic, Pessimistic, Trusting, and Envious (Poncela-Casasnovas et al., 2016). Can you guess which personality type is the most common? Surprisingly, Envious is the most common personality type, with 30 percent of the share, pessimistic, trusting, and optimistic scoring 20 percent. The remaining 10 percent of people were categorized into a fifth group that could not be defined. The researchers compiled the responses of 541 volunteers on questions regarding hundreds of social dilemmas. They had options ranging from collaborating or engaging in conflict with others based on their individual or collective interests.

Suppose your loved one with dementia used to be optimistic and always cheerful before they developed dementia. In that case, they can have the darker side of their personality become more apparent than before as the disease progresses. They could become more aggressive, anxious, and agitated at the early stages of dementia and physically and emotionally abusive and distrustful in the middle to late stages of dementia because of the changes in their brain due to the disease.

DEMENTIA AND CHANGES IN BEHAVIOR: A REVIEW

In the middle and late stages of most dementia-related conditions, it is normal to notice the person starting to behave differently (NHS, 2021). It can be distressing to witness your loved one act differently than how you know them to behave. It can also be just as distressing for the person to see themselves become someone they are not and start behaving differently than before. As the disease resulting in the person's dementia begins to progress, they can experience behavioral changes that other people find challenging to comprehend. That can be the case if they do not know what is going on regarding the symptoms that become apparent in the different stages of dementia. It is arguably one of the most challenging aspects of living with dementia for both the person diagnosed with the condition and those caring for them. Several reasons can explain the behavioral changes the person is going through, such as:

- They may be frustrated or fearful about how dementia changes their lives and affects their cognitive functioning, such as memory loss or language problems.
- They may be experiencing challenges regarding their mental and physical health.
- They may be experiencing problems with orientation. For example, they may not know what year, month, day, or time it is, or they may not remember places and people they regularly visit and interact with.
- The quality of time and contact they spend with others may be reduced, or people do not want to be around them as much.
- If the place where they are staying is too dark (i.e., has limited natural light coming through the windows), they may become confused and distressed because they may not be able to figure out where they are.
- Feeling like they have lost control of themselves, they may be frustrated with how other people behave toward them or feel like no one is listening to or understanding them.

GENERAL TIPS: FOLLOW THE P.E.E.L METHOD

The P.E.E.L method is a practical way to understand and manage undesirable and problematic behaviors when interacting with your loved one with dementia. Sometimes when you are in a difficult or uncomfortable situation, it can be challenging to think about what to do to manage the situation with careful consideration of what your loved one is experiencing emotionally. There is a way to get around this respectfully. Below are general tips to follow to manage problem behaviors thoughtfully (Budson, 2022):

- **Provide reassurance**: Your loved one with dementia may experience challenges with interacting with the world around them due to their memory loss. They may not recognize people and things that were once familiar to them. They may have difficulty understanding noise, crowds, and different activities happening around them and can quickly feel overwhelmed. They can even get worried or terrified when they cannot see you for even a few minutes when you have gone out together to the shops, for instance. In their mind, they may think you have been gone for hours. Several reasons can explain why your loved one with dementia may feel more worried or terrified, especially if they have never experienced these emotions before to the degree they are feeling them now.

Remind yourself whenever they are yelling or feeling irritated with whatever is happening; it may be related to their fear or anxiety. Use phrases such as "Everything is all right," "You are not alone," and "There is no need to worry" to reassure them that you are there for them and everything is fine. It can also help to provide comfort and help reduce or stop some of their problem behaviors. You may need to reassure them continuously.

- **Exercise empathy**: It is essential to look at things from your loved one's point of view. How you think your loved one is experiencing things can be strikingly different from how they are actually experiencing them. For example, your loved one gets angry when the nurse comes to help with maintaining their hygiene in the comfort of their home. It may not be easy to understand why they feel that way, but thinking about things from their perspective can help explain it. They may perceive the nurse as a stranger because of their memory loss, despite the nurse helping them for a long time. They may not remember needing help to take care of their hygiene.

From their perspective, they think a stranger is asking them to sit down at the dressing table to trim their nails to keep them short and clean; of course, your loved one would feel anxious or confused. Would you not feel the same way? Rethinking things from the perspective of your loved one with dementia can help improve your ability to empathize with them. It can give you clues figuring out how best to manage their problem behavior.

- **Engage in something else to distract them**: Never tell your loved one to stop a problem behavior because that hardly ever works. So, turning their attention to something fun they enjoy to do often works best. Why do you think that may be? When distracted by something they like doing or find interesting, it takes them away from the problem behavior or the stressful environment. It forces them to focus on something else. There are many ways to distract your loved one. So, you could take your loved one into another room, start engaging them in a random conversation or activity, point out something intriguing, or give them a beloved object. Also, while distracting them, use a gentle touch and tone of voice to de-escalate the behavior calmly.
- **Look out for your non-verbal communication cues**: As the disease progresses, their abilities diminish, and your loved one may rely on their caregiver to interpret and understand what is happening around them. Consciously or subconsciously, they may regulate their emotions

according to how they feel. For instance, if you feel angry and upset because of their behavior or something else unrelated to them, they will also start feeling just as angry and upset as you are. Even if you are using reassuring words at the moment, your loved one can still pick up from your tone of voice or body language that you are feeling angry and upset. So, it is crucial to stay calm and relaxed, but also you must pay attention to and be mindful of your non-verbal communication when faced with problem behavior.

SPECIFIC TIPS FOR THE MOST COMMON BEHAVIOR CHANGES

As the disease progresses, your loved one will experience specific behavioral changes, which can be challenging. Always keep in the back of your mind that their behavior change is never deliberate. Below are some practical tips and advice to help you manage their shift in behavior thoughtfully (Alzheimer's Association, n.d.e.; Better Health, 2014a; Hobson, 2023; Smith et al., 2023):

Repetition or Repetitive Behavior

- Be considerate and patient.
- Assist your loved one in finding the answer themselves.

- Look for an explanation, such as the person feeling out of place, and use reassuring words.
- Offer general reassurance; for instance, you could tell them, "You do not need to worry about that as everything is under control."
- Encourage your loved one to talk about something they enjoyed, such as an event they liked going to or a period of time in their youth they were most happy.
- Turn the behavior into an activity. For example, if they are asking you questions repeatedly, you could turn that into a game of 30 seconds, whereby you get to ask each other simple questions, and the other person must answer each question in 30 seconds.
- Utilize memory aids.

Aggressiveness and Anger

- Refrain from confronting the person or talking about the angry behavior because it will be counterproductive.
- Do not physically touch them during the angry behavior.
- Let your loved one express the aggression they are feeling inside.
- Turn their attention to a more pleasurable, enjoyable, or exciting activity.

- Identify patterns in the aggression or the immediate cause of the aggression.
- Seek help from other people during the outburst.
- Never take the outbursts of anger personally—you are not to blame.
- Control your feelings of anger. Be positive and give reassurance. Speak in a gentle tone of voice.
- Have minimal distractions. Evaluate your loved one's environment and make changes to avoid situations that could anger them.
- Take a timeout. If your loved one's surroundings are safe and you can take a break, take that moment to gather yourself.
- Ensure you and your loved one with dementia are safe.

Hallucinations

- Be reassuring and give a simple answer to any allegations. Refrain from arguing or reasoning with them to show them that their accusations or suspicions are baseless.
- Turn their attention to another activity, such as taking a stroll.
- Give honest responses.
- Make changes to the environment as needed.

Suspicions and Delusions

- Do not bear a grudge against what they are saying.
- Refrain from arguing or trying to convince them otherwise.
- Give a simple response.
- Distract them with something else to occupy their mind.
- Make an exact copy of any lost items.

Wandering and Restlessness

- Ensure your loved one has enough food and something to drink.
- Have a daily routine, including daily brain exercises.
- Consider going with them on a walk to the shops or installing tracking devices and alarm systems, such as telecare, ensuring they are always safe.
- If they tend to fidget quite a bit, give them something to hold in their hands.
- At the time of day when your loved one is most likely to start wandering off, you can distract them with a fun activity.
- Eliminate noise and confusion.
- Consider installing child-safety devices in the house to secure all windows and doors.

- Keep items your loved one would want if they were to leave the house, such as handbags, shoes, keys, or sunglasses.
- Look for comfortable chairs that restrict movement because that can make it challenging for your loved one to get up without any help. When you find these chairs, consider buying them for your loved one to prevent them from wandering off.
- Make your neighbors and local police aware of your loved one's wandering tendencies, and give them your contact number.
- Have your loved one wear clothes with identifying labels or a bracelet with their ID. Also, many digital devices in the market use GPS technology, which you can purchase to help track your loved one's whereabouts.
- If you call for a police search to be done, have a recently taken photograph of your loved one and some clothing you have not washed for secure-and-rescue dogs to sniff to try to find them.
- Arrange an appointment with the doctor as disorientation could be one of the side effects of the medication they are consuming, drug interactions, or over-medicating.

Hiding and Hoarding Things

- Look for your loved one's usual hiding places and evaluate these first when things go missing in the house.
- Provide your loved one with a chest of drawers full of random and odd items for them to sort out, as this can satisfy the need to keep busy.
- Ensure your loved one can find their way around their environment because if they struggle to recognize where they are, that may add to their hoarding tendencies.

Sleeping Difficulties and Sundowning

- Sundowning is the disruption of the sleep-wake cycle. People living with dementia can experience wakefulness, disorientation, and confusion at sunset and throughout the night (Smith et al., 2023).
- Make improvements to sleep hygiene.
- Ensure a night light is always on in their room.
- Place a chamber pot near their bed to make it easier to relieve themselves at night.
- Engage your loved one in moderate to intense physical activity to help them sleep better at night.
- Keep tabs on their napping during the afternoon.
- Limit your loved one's caffeine, sugar, and unhealthy food intake during the day.

SUMMARY

- A study on human behavior conducted in 2016 discovered four basic personality types: Optimistic, pessimistic, trusting, and envious. They found that the most common personality type was envious, followed by the other personality types, which scored the same. The changes in the brain of someone with dementia can cause them to experience personality changes that go from their baseline personality, for instance, optimistic in the early stages of dementia, to abusive and distrustful in the late stages of the disease.
- As the disease progresses from the early, middle, to late stages of dementia, it can become distressing for the person with dementia and those caring for them when their behavior changes. Also, it can be challenging to understand, and there are many reasons for the significant changes in behavior. Those can vary from frustration or fear about the progression of the disease, their mental and physical health, problems with their physical surroundings and orientation, reduced contact with other people, or feeling not listened to or misunderstood.
- Generally, you can follow the steps described in the PE.E.L method to manage the problem behaviors of your loved one, such as providing reassurance, exercising empathy by looking at things from your

loved one's point of view, engaging your loved one in something else to distract them, and looking out for your non-verbal communication cues.
- When your loved one begins to exhibit behavioral changes, it is essential to remember that they are not deliberately exhibiting these behaviors. People living with dementia experience these common behavior changes as the disease progresses: Repetition or repetitive behavior, aggressiveness and anger, hallucinations, suspicions and delusions, wandering and restlessness, hiding and hoarding things, sleep difficulties, and sundowning. The underlying themes of the practical tips and advice shared to manage these common behavior changes are: Offering reassurance, staying calm and patient, thinking ahead to prevent a similar situation from happening again, controlling your negative emotions, and studying their usual behavior patterns.

It is never easy when a loved one begins to change as a result of the development of dementia. However, with the proper knowledge and support, you can immensely make their situation more manageable. Adapting the same mindset to other aspects of your loved one's everyday life—such as bathing, eating, sleeping, and exercising—will also significantly help them.

The next chapter discusses ways in which you can help your loved one maintain physical health and well-being despite their condition.

8

IMPROVING DAILY LIFE AMID DEMENTIA

As previously mentioned in an earlier chapter, various types of dementia affect different parts of the brain and have different symptoms from one another. These other types of dementia are Alzheimer's disease, Vascular dementia, Lewy body dementia, Frontotemporal lobe dementia, and mixed dementia. Among the many changes in emotion and behavior, cognitive decline, needing care and support from caregivers and family members, and other things people with dementia experience, there is growing evidence that reveals this population can have an eating and swallowing disorder known as dysphagia. The National Institutes of Health has stated that nearly 45 percent of people diagnosed with dementia and other dementia-related conditions experience swallowing problems (National Foundation of Swallowing Disorders, 2017). As the disease progresses and becomes severe for those diagnosed with dementia, this percentage increases. For example, 80 percent of older people diagnosed with dementia in care facilities have some degree of dysphagia.

The development of dysphagia can be dangerous, especially if the area of the swallowing problem is not detected and the underlying cause is untreated. When people living with dementia develop dysphagia, and it is untreated, it can lead to serious health problems, such as weight loss, malnutrition, and dehydration. These are manageable health problems. However, even manageable health problems can lead to other significantly severe health problems in senior citizens depending on their age, medical history, comorbidities, lifestyle habits, and mental and physical health state. For example, the development of dysphagia can lead to serious lung-related health complications, such as aspiration pneumonia, which may necessitate the person to be hospitalized and even threaten their life. When all these factors are combined, they can give rise to loneliness, isolation, and a depressive mood, and they may not even want to seek medical assistance and not eat anything because of the difficulty of swallowing food and the other symptoms they have from their underlying condition, i.e., dementia. Dysphagia has a negative impact on the person's overall quality of life. However, there is hope at the end of this tunnel. When people with dementia treat their dysphagia, it can help relieve the symptoms of their underlying condition, such as dementia and other dementia-related conditions (Microsoft

Start, n.d.). Thus, caregivers and family members play a crucial role in helping to identify swallowing problems in their loved ones with dementia and encouraging them to follow medical advice on suitable treatment, such as oral intake.

PERSONAL HYGIENE

Within the stages of dementia, your loved one will need your help taking care of themselves, including keeping themselves clean. Keep in mind that they may feel frustrated and embarrassed, or they may even reject your help. Below are some practical tips to help you to support your loved one in taking care of their everyday life activities (Alzheimer's Association, n.d.g; Alzheimer's Society, 2021d; Alzheimer's Society, 2021e; Better Health, 2014c; National Institute on Aging, 2017):

Bathing

- Give them privacy during washing and dressing times.
- Make changes to the environment to accommodate their bathing needs.
- Create daily routines to help with bathing, such as choosing the optimal time of the day to help them bathe or when your loved one feels most relaxed every day.

- Simplify bathing. For example, you could consider sponge baths that do not require submersion or shower spray to clean.
- Make preparations in advance for bath time.
- Help your loved one to feel in control of bathing. Expanding on the earlier example of the sponge bath, you could give them a sponge to clean their arms and torso while you clean their back.
- Respect your loved one's dignity.
- Use a nurturing touch to make bathing soothing.
- Be flexible.

Toileting

- Remove obstructions to get to the bathroom.
- Offer reminders, such as putting an A4 laminated sign that says, "Remember to wash your hands after using the toilet."
- Monitor their consistency regarding bowel movements.
- Consider having products that can assist with constipation in the house. If the need arises, you will be prepared to handle this problem.
- Show them your support.

Dressing

- Make dressing simpler. For example, you could give your loved one two options to decide which shoes or pants they want to wear.
- Make the activity of getting dressed organized and fun to do.
- Select clothing items for your loved ones that are comfortable and simple.
- Be flexible.

Dental Care

- Give short and simple instructions to take care of their oral hygiene.
- Use a "watch me" or a "hand-over-hand" method to ensure your loved one is brushing their teeth correctly, or you could do it for them.
- Monitor your loved one's daily dental care.
- Help your loved one keep up with visiting the dentist regularly for as long as possible.
- When making the appointment on behalf of your loved one, it is always best practice to advise the dentist that the patient has dementia and they may be unable to cooperate.

NUTRITION

It is usual to think about memory loss, difficulty finding the right words, disorientation, or poor executive functioning skills when it comes to dementia. These cognitive functioning skills are central to dementia and other dementia-related conditions. Nonetheless, there are other difficulties in caring for your loved one with dementia that involves helping them manage their everyday life activities, such as eating, drinking, bathing, dressing, and exercising. Also, that includes difficulty with eating and changes in appetite, which often results in unintentional weight loss. A study published in *Alzheimer's & Dementia: A Journal of the Alzheimer's Association* had over 16 000 adult participants and found a strong correlation between unexpected weight loss and dementia severity. Adequate nutrition is vital for everyone to maintain good health. It is even more imperative for people with dementia who could have difficulties with eating to receive adequate nutrition. People living with dementia may find it difficult to consume food because of the following reasons (Agespace, n.d.; Alzheimer's Association, n.d.f.; Heerema, 2020; Hill, 2022c; WebMD Editorial Contributors, 2022):

- Loss of appetite.
- No longer recognizing the food you may place on their plate.

- Having dentures that do not fit properly or lack of healthy teeth.
- Side effects of new medications, such as incontinence and changes in taste.
- Lack of physical activity could be affecting their appetite.
- Feeling overwhelmed with too many food choices.
- Memory loss could have caused your loved one to forget how to chew and swallow food, move food to their mouth, or use utensils.
- Problems with judgment.
- Distracted by their environment.
- Decreased sense of vision, smell, and taste.
- Depression or anxiety can cause people not to want to eat.
- Unfamiliar pain in the body, particularly in the teeth and gums, can make someone lose their appetite.
- Fatigue.
- Lack of muscle movement.
- Chewing and swallowing changes, such as storing food in their cheeks.
- A new health condition or illness that is worsening, such as a cold, stomach problem, chronic illness, or incontinence, can make someone not want to eat or even drink fewer fluids.

Tips to Help Them Eat and Drink Safely

- Provide a well-balanced diet with different food groups, such as vegetables, fruits, whole grains, dairy products, and protein foods.
- Minimize consumption of foods with high saturated fat and cholesterol. Some fat is needed in the body to maintain good health. However, not all fats are good. So, limit your loved one's intake that can cause bad health, for example, butter and fatty cuts of muscle meat.
- Limit foods with refined sugars, commonly found in processed foods that contain more calories than vitamins, minerals, and fiber. You can trick your sweet tooth into enjoying healthier food options still packed with sugar, such as fruit or juice-sweetened pastries. Surprisingly, if in the middle to late stages of dementia, your loved one has a loss of appetite, adding sugar to whatever food they eat could encourage eating.
- Reduce foods with high sodium, which often results in high blood pressure. Spices and herbs are great alternatives to sodium to season food.
- Encourage your loved one to drink fluids. Sometimes dementia and other dementia-related conditions can affect a person's ability to recognize they are thirsty. So, it is crucial to encourage your

loved one to drink fluids frequently. If they have difficulty swallowing water, try giving them fruit or vegetable juice, soup, or yogurt, which all contain water. Also, you can try giving them liquids that are thickened by adding cornstarch or unflavored gelatin. Other drinks that count toward liquid intake are tea and coffee.
- Eliminate distractions to help your loved one concentrate on eating the meal you have prepared for them.
- Choose soft foods that are easy to swallow, such as pudding, steamed vegetables, salad greens, canned fruit, and mashed potatoes. Also, bite-size and finger foods, such as fish fingers, chicken nuggets, and tuna sandwiches, can work too. If your loved one cannot eat solid foods anymore, masking up or pureeing the food in a blender can help.
- Be flexible with food preferences and how much food they want to eat. Sometimes people with late-stage dementia and other dementia-related conditions tend to eat more when offered smaller meals or snacks during the day rather than having three large meals. Essentially, take every opportunity to find what they find acceptable.
- Provide enough time to eat because it might take them longer to eat during the late stage of dementia and other dementia-related conditions.

- Eat together because social interaction can encourage your loved one to eat.
- Encourage independence by adapting serving dishes and utensils and demonstrating eating behavior to allow your loved one to feed themselves as much as possible during meals. Be ready to help when your loved one needs it.
- Look out for signs of choking during meals. Get lessons on the Heimlich maneuver (abdominal thrusts) in case of a choking emergency.

EXERCISE

Eating healthy and maintaining an active lifestyle is good for everyone. It is even more imperative for people with dementia and other dementia-related conditions. As the disease gradually worsens, finding ways for your loved one living with dementia to eat healthy foods and maintain an active lifestyle may become challenging as time progresses. Below are some practical tips and advice that may help (National Institute on Aging, n.d.):

General Tips

- Help your loved one get started with an activity or join them in their fun to make it more enjoyable. People with dementia can have little to no interest or may not take the initiative and can have difficulty starting a new activity. However, you can change this

by doing the planning as that can encourage them to join the activity.
- Include music in the exercise routine or activities if you know it will motivate your loved one. Also, you could dance to the music where possible.
- Consider how much activity your loved one can do at one time. It may be best to engage them in numerous short "mini-workouts" rather than hours of exercise.
- Take a walk together every day. Keeping an active lifestyle is good for caregivers, too!

Suggested Activities for Early to Middle Stages of Dementia

Below is a list of some exercises to engage your loved one in the early to middle stages of dementia. Also, any form of exercise can bring health benefits. The examples are the following (Alzheimer's Society, n.d.b, nd.c.):

- **Gardening**: It is a physical activity that encourages people to get outdoors and can be enjoyable for people at any stage of dementia. Gardening is an activity that can be varied according to the level of intensity your loved one enjoys. For example, if they enjoy something moderate, they could do weeding or pruning. If they enjoy something more intense, they could engage in raking or mowing the grass. These gardening activities can improve muscle strength and breathing.

- **Indoor bowling**: If your loved one enjoys indoor bowling, they could continue doing it or start to engage in a new ball game. Some community leisure centers have bowling centers that offer sessions, or you could purchase sets from toy or sports shops.
- **Dance**: Like gardening, dancing can vary from group sessions to balls. Dancing is a fun social activity and a great way to engage in some exercise. Also, dancing can increase strength and flexibility, help your loved one stay agile, and reduce stress.
- **Seated exercises**: Seated exercises are an excellent idea at home or in a local class with others. These exercises are aimed at building or maintaining muscle strength and balance. The instructor usually demonstrates the seated exercises at least once to help people to know how to do the exercises. These exercises can form part of a regular or developing program for people with dementia. Below is not an exhaustive list of seated exercises:
- Marching.
- Twisting the upper body from left to right and vice versa.
- Moving the toes up and down.
- Raising the arms to the ceiling.
- Raising the opposite leg and arm at the same time.
- Bending the legs.
- Clapping below the legs.
- Moving the legs in a cycling motion.

- Moving the arms in a circular motion.
- Standing up and sitting down from the chair.
- **Swimming**: Swimming is an excellent activity for people with dementia, as it can be soothing and calming to be in the water. However, it must be under supervision. Also, swimming can improve balance and reduce the possibility of frequent falling in older people.
- **Tai chi or qigong**: Tai chi and qigong are a series of integrated, simple physical movements and meditation, or otherwise, they are known to be Chinese martial arts that can help with improving balance and stability, staying agile, and reducing the risk of frequent falls in older people.
- **Walking**: Anyone can engage in walking no matter their fitness level. It is free, requires no equipment, and people can walk anywhere. You can help determine the suitable distance and time your loved one can spend walking according to their fitness level. Alternatively, you could find organizations that do group walks in the community, which involve a walk leader and various distances.

Suggested Activities for Late Stage of Dementia

- When getting up or going to bed while seated, drag your body along the edge of the bed from one end to the other. This exercise helps strengthen the

muscles that help with getting up from a chair or a bed.
- Balance in a standing position can form part of day-to-day activities, such as showering or washing the dishes. It can help with balance and posture.
- Sit unsupported for a couple of minutes every day. This activity helps to maintain strong stomach and back muscles. Someone must always be there to assist because of the risk of falling while doing this exercise.
- Stand up and move around regularly, which can help to maintain strong leg muscles and good balance.

SUMMARY

- People with dementia can develop a swallowing problem, known as dysphagia, as the disease severity progresses. Dysphagia, when left untreated, can lead to serious health problems and, when treated, can help relieve symptoms of dementia and other dementia-related conditions. Caregivers and family members play a significant role in helping their loved ones to identify swallowing problems and following treatment.
- People with dementia can have many reasons for having difficulty eating, ranging from loss of appetite, depression or anxiety, and chewing and

swallowing changes, such as storing food in their cheeks.
- There are several ways to help them to eat and drink safely, such as providing a variety of foods, limiting distractions, and eating together.
- Different ways of maintaining personal hygiene were shared that can be used in any stage of dementia.
- To encourage your loved one to exercise to maintain an active lifestyle and stay healthy, you could get them started on one activity or do it with them, add music to the sessions, be reasonable about how much activity they can get in at once, and walk together daily.
- People in the early to middle stages of dementia can engage in these exercises to maintain good health: Gardening, indoor bowling, dance, seated exercises, swimming, tai chi or qigong, and walking.
- People in the late stage of dementia can engage in these exercises to maintain good health, such as when getting up or going to bed while seated, they can drag their body from one end to the other, balance in a standing position, sit unsupported for a couple of minutes daily, and stand up and move around regularly.

Caring for your loved one with dementia does not always have to be a struggle. There are still plenty of activities that you and your loved one can enjoy, keep your mind off the stress, and, most of all, boost your relationship.

The next chapter will offer simple activities that will benefit your loved one's mental and physical health, and further deepen your relationship while dealing with dementia.

9

STRENGTHENING YOUR BOND

Did you know a study found that having a close relationship with a caregiver can slow down a dementia patient's decline? A study led by John Hopkins and Utah State University published in *The Journal of Gerontology Series B: Psychological Sciences and Social Sciences* has shown that the patient-caregiver relationship can have a direct influence on how dementia and other dementia-related conditions progress in a patient (Johns Hopkins Medical Institutions, 2009). Patients received surveys to complete and choose statements most fitting to their situation. They had to rate their level of agreement or disagreement with six statements. Some of those statements read as the following: "My relationship with the care recipient is close," "The care recipient makes me feel like a special person," and "The care recipient and I can always discuss things together." Their results were interesting. The patients who felt they were close with their caregiver scored highly on cognitive tests throughout the study compared to those patients who had a distant relationship with their caregiver.

The positive effect was that the level of closeness the patient had to their caregiver was significantly more when that caregiver was a spouse compared to any family member. The Mini-Mental State Exam was one of the cognitive tests used in the study. Also, when the patient was close to their caregiver, they scored highly on a functional test known as the *Clinical Dementia Rating*. They remained very close to the baseline as time progressed compared to the patients who were more distant from their caregivers.

WHAT TO CONSIDER WHEN COMING UP WITH ACTIVITIES FOR YOUR LOVED ONE

People living with dementia or other dementia-related conditions want to have a connection with the people who care for them. Also, they want to feel fulfilled, just like everybody else. Engaging your loved one in a number of stimulating, exciting, fun, creative, and meaningful ways to enjoy the time spent with their loved ones would be worthwhile for them.

You may be asking yourself what you should consider when creating activities for your loved one. Generally, choosing the appropriate activities for your loved one with dementia is a personal choice and should be based on your loved one's interests and abilities. Engaging your loved one in a number of daily activities can be helpful in the early stages of their dementia to give them structure, and a routine that incorporates fun activities will benefit them. Below are a few pointers that you could consider when selecting your activities (Craig, 2021; Senior Services of America, 2022):

- **Timing is everything**: If you want to ensure success in the activities you want to do with your loved one with dementia, the timing has to be right. People living with dementia can be unpredictable. So, prepare yourself to exercise flexibility and patience with everything concerning them and in activities with them. Pay close attention to or remember when your loved one seemed joyous, fulfilled, distracted, anxious, or irritable. Ensure that your loved one is not distracted by anything so they can focus solely on the stimulating activity you have planned for them.
- **Choose frustration and failure-free activities**: Whenever you are planning activities with your loved one with dementia, always seek to pick activities that they will be able to do, have simple and easy-to-follow steps, and an activity they can complete without feeling frustrated or upset. If you know of some activities your loved one has enjoyed in the past, you can stick to those and adjust the

skills to match the ability level of your loved one as needed. There are a few ways you can support your loved one through the activity, such as helping them with parts of the activity they are struggling with doing themselves, helping them to focus on one particular task at a time of the activity, and never correcting them.

- **Activities must be energizing**: It is always good to have people living with dementia remain active physically and mentally as much as they can to keep their minds and senses energized. A fantastic way to keep them physically and mentally active would be to pay attention to the activities your loved one enjoys doing or activities they have previously enjoyed. For example, if they have always owned a dog, they may enjoy having a stuffed dog to care for and have as a companion. Generally, you can encourage your loved one to get involved with the day-to-day activities, such as folding the laundry and putting it in the chest of drawers or wardrobes. It can help them feel a sense of accomplishment.

SUGGESTED ACTIVITIES

Creative Activities

- **Knitting or crocheting**: To engage your loved one in making a homemade quilt, you may need to put a skein of yarn in their hands to spark their interest (Samuels, 2023). Alternatively, let them familiarize themselves with the weight of the yarn and the scratchiness of it. If they have some prior experience of being able to knit or crochet a little bit, their muscle memory could remind them of how to knit or crochet, even if they may have mild to severe memory decline.

- **Music**: If your loved one with dementia used to play an instrument or loved listening to or playing music, you could introduce them to playing simple instruments or singing their favorite songs. If your loved one has mild cognitive deterioration, music ability can be their strongest cognitive ability above other memory functions.
- **Painting or arts and crafts**: Painting and arts and crafts are a safe way to encourage your loved one to express their feelings creatively. It is a great idea to encourage them to use bold, bright colors on large surfaces and use rolls of butcher paper to have them create art without the stress of creating a masterpiece.
- **Making collages**: Cut out images of memories in magazines or newspapers. You can select magazines that reflect some of the memories you have shared with them or those under the subjects that fit your loved one's desires or things they like, such as cooking, travel, fashion, gardening, or dancing.

Another idea would be to scan and print colored copies of old family pictures to create scrapbook pages.

Fulfilling Activities

- **Puzzles**: Select puzzles for your loved one with large, tactile pieces because it stimulates the brain to focus on the size and texture. Also, as your loved one actively holds the large, tactile pieces and tries to put the puzzle pieces together, they use their short-term memory. So, engaging in puzzles every day will improve their short-term and long-term memory. Another idea is to give them wooden color or shape puzzles to put together, as they can be easier to match and are safe for your loved one, especially if your loved one is frail.
- **Folding laundry**: If you care for a senior woman, laundry may be a familiar activity for them. Your loved one can find soft fabrics and the repeated motion of folding clothes calming. Also, certain detergent smells could elicit beautiful memories for your loved one. You could start with simple items, such as T-shirts and socks. However, do not give them fitted sheets and buttoned shirts because your loved one could find such items challenging to fold.
- **Handy tasks**: If your loved one enjoyed repairing things, you could suggest a task with visible results.

Also, if they have a high motor function, you could engage them in painting wooden boards or putting together PVC pipes for the plumbing system. If they have advanced dementia, you could engage them in wooden or plastic vintage tinker play tool sets.

- **Managing knots**: Your loved one may enjoy tying loose knots or untying them. You could do this along with a thick rope. Alternatively, you could make the knots and have them untie the knots. However, do not make the knots too tight, or have your loved one use a rough rope.

Sensory Activities

- **Explore nature**: For example, smelling flowers (and other objects) can elicit more vivid emotional memories than photographs. Our brains use the hippocampus and the amygdala to process smells, the same brain centers that control memories. Familiar smells, such as your loved one's favorite flowers or freshly baked cookies, can elicit positive emotions. Conversely, it is essential to help your loved one avoid smells that can cause them anxiety, such as diesel fuel or gunpowder, that could be associated with a traumatic event like an accident or a violent home invasion.
- **Explore familiar objects**: Tactile stimulation from familiar objects can elicit memories in a way that

pictures or verbal prompting cannot do. For example, if your loved one does not remember their first graduation or wedding, the feeling of a graduation gown or a white-looking veil could elicit memories.

- **Taste familiar food and drinks**: Similar to smells, the taste of familiar food and drinks can elicit memories and emotions. For example, your loved one's favorite vanilla cake or a home-cooked meal could bring back celebratory memories, such as birthdays, wedding ceremonies, or happy dinners; a sip of coffee or tea could recall quiet and peaceful mornings on vacation.
- **Feel different textures**: Feeling different textures can stimulate the senses and give memory cues. If your loved one with dementia loves pets, you can provide an animal for your loved one to feel their soft fur. Also, you can consider damp soil or leaves if they love gardening. You can also use textures to complete specific tasks. For example, if you want to sort out different fabrics for laundry, you could have your loved one sort them by touch.

Technology-based Activities

Technology use can have a wide range of health and safety benefits that are surprising for people with dementia. Immersive technology, such as virtual reality, can provide them with sensory and visual stimulation that can improve cognitive functioning in the comfort of their home. Below are some suggestions for technology-based activities:

- **Explore places with live streams and sites like Google Earth**: Nature reserve parks and aquariums worldwide offer live internet streams for people who love animals. Art museums, such as the Louvre in Paris, offer live tours of their beautiful galleries that can last for hours. Since it shows various images continuously, the live streams can provide your loved one with visual stimulation, especially if your loved one often stays home.

Google Earth is another tremendous immersive technology, as your loved one can see photographs from around the world. For instance, if you have pictures of different places your loved one loves, from their childhood camping site or the Nile River—you could upload the pictures into Google Earth for them to explore.

- **Create a family video**: Technology helps families to stay connected via phone calls, video calls, and chats. However, if relatives did not have the time to talk, having their presence on video calls, for instance, can be comforting. Encourage family members and friends to record videos of themselves, upload them onto a tablet, and play them when your loved one feels restless or has trouble sleeping. If tablets do not work for your loved one, you could take the videos to an electronics shop and ask them to upload them onto a DVD.

Other Activities

- **Do something outside**: Take your loved one for a walk, plant flowers, feed birds, or go to the park (Stringfellow, 2019). Ensure they are going to a safe environment to get in some exercise, reconnect with mother nature, have their skins absorb a little vitamin D, and meet new people.
- **Visit a zoo**: A day at the zoo or farm can be fulfilling and rewarding for children and adults. Also, who does not like animals? It can be very beneficial for lowering blood pressure and boosting serotonin levels to take a trip to the zoo or a farm where your loved one can touch and communicate with animals.
- **Prepare afternoon tea**: It can be helpful to enjoy some tea outdoors and take in the activity of others and the changes of sun, shade, and clouds; seeing the growth of plants and experiencing wildlife can benefit your loved one with dementia. All you need to make this happen is to create a safe space with a secure garden to sit in, enjoy a cup of tea, and hold a lovely conversation.

SUMMARY

- People with dementia who have a close relationship with a caregiver can slow down their cognitive decline compared to those who may have a distant relationship with their caregiver. Also, if the caregiver is a spouse compared to a family member or friend, that can significantly result in better functionality and cognitive functioning.
- People with dementia and other dementia-related conditions want to connect with others and feel fulfilled, just like everybody else. You can engage your loved one with dementia in a number of stimulating, fun, creative, and meaningful activities when spending time with them. However, you must consider things before engaging your loved one in activities, such as ensuring the timing is right, choosing frustration and failure-free activities, and the activities must be energizing.
- Some suggested creative activities were knitting or crocheting, listening to or playing music, painting or arts and crafts, and making collages.
- Fulfilling activities suggested for people with dementia were puzzles, folding laundry, handy tasks, and managing knots to encourage visual and tactile stimulation.
- Sensory activities suggested are exploring nature and familiar objects, tasting familiar food and drinks, and

feeling different textures to elicit memories and emotions and stimulate the senses.
- Technology-based activities suggested for people with dementia are exploring places through live streams and sites like Google Earth and creating a family video because they can encourage visual stimulation and help keep your loved one connected with their family and friends via phone or video calls, which can be comforting.
- Other suggested activities for people with dementia that can benefit their mind and body are doing something outside, visiting a zoo or farm, and preparing afternoon tea.

The activities suggested in this chapter are for people with dementia to help them benefit from the activities in numerous ways and for you. After all, taking care of your loved one with dementia can be so stressful and draining. In the next chapter, you will learn more about the importance of ensuring that your health and well-being remain intact. More specifically, you will explore practical techniques that caregivers can adopt to avoid suffering from caregiver burnout.

10

TAKING CARE OF YOURSELF

Caring for yourself is like putting an oxygen mask on airplanes (Family Advisory Board of the Transitions ACR, 2019). Before the airplane takes off, flight attendants give instructions to passengers to inform them of what to do in case of an emergency. One of the instructions flight attendants tell passengers is to put their oxygen masks on first before they think of helping other people, even if it is children. Because if they run out of oxygen, they will not be able to help other people, even their loved ones. It is true when it pertains to self-care because taking care of yourself first is a priority, not a selfish act. Taking care of someone with a mental health condition is challenging, and taking some time for yourself is vital. It can start with 5 minutes per day!

When you practice self-care, you can feel relaxed, more grounded, energized, and healthier, experience better sleep, eat better, manage relationships thoughtfully, experience less anxiety or fewer negative thoughts, and feel better able to manage challenges.

Self-care will look different for everyone, and what works for you may not work for your family member, but what it does to your body and mind matters the most. It benefits your physical, mental, and spiritual health and can support your daily functioning. Making time for self-care may be difficult, but it is an investment toward your health and well-being. Building new habits or routines takes time. Research suggests that building a new habit into your daily routine takes at least two months. Keep at it. The same study has revealed that missing a day of self-care will not affect your progress toward making self-care a habit and priority.

WHAT IS CAREGIVER BURNOUT?

Caregiver burnout is when one feels physically, emotionally, and mentally exhausted (Cleveland Clinic, 2019). Many caregivers, when they experience burnout, can change their attitude, from positive and nurturing to negative and not caring about anything. Burnout can occur when caregivers do not receive the support they need or if they try to go beyond their breaking point physically or mentally. Many caregivers can feel guilty when they spend time caring for themselves instead of caring for their loved ones with dementia. Stressed caregivers who are "burned out" can experience fatigue, anxiety, and depression. That can feel like an extended period where numbness, panic, or sadness can start, and the mind convinces you that trying to improve your predicament would be pointless (Lawler, 2023).

There is no doubt that caregiving can be strenuous and, at the same time, can be tremendously rewarding. Caregivers need to seek support from family members, close friends, or organizations that specialize in adult social care to help lessen the burden of caring for their loved one with dementia by themselves. That will, hopefully, make them feel less alone and appreciated in their role (Cohen, 2022).

SYMPTOMS OF CAREGIVER BURNOUT

Caregiver burnout is associated with isolation and feeling discouraged. It can be challenging to recognize it, especially if this is the first time you have experienced it. Some of the symptoms that someone could be experiencing caregiver burnout are the following (Lawler, 2023):

- Caregivers can experience a change in their attitude. They can go from loving and caring to disheartened and not caring as much.
- Social withdrawal from the people who love you the most, such as family and friends.
- Losing interest and pleasure in activities and things you previously enjoyed.
- Feeling pettish, hopeless, helpless, and tired.

- A change in eating habits and concerning weight loss.
- Different sleeping behavior. A study published in the Journal of Gerontological Nursing in May 2020 found that caregivers of people living with dementia, particularly their family members with dementia, had trouble falling asleep and experienced lower sleep quality.
- Having a compromised immune system that causes them to feel under the weather or get sick more often than before. When this happens, caring for a loved one with dementia can leave you feeling further depleted than ever before.
- Getting irritated easily.

TIPS TO MANAGE CAREGIVER BURNOUT

If you feel like caregiver burnout is something you are going through, there are practical steps that you can take to overcome it. You must learn to set boundaries and limits that will honor you and your caregiving responsibilities. Below are some things that can help (Alzheimer's Association, n.d.h; Lawler, 2023: Mayo Clinic, 2022; Robinson et al., 2023; Smith, 2023):

- **Prioritize self-care**: Find what works for you and make time to do those things. For example, you could go on daily walks to get away from your situation for a couple of minutes. Also, practicing mindfulness can help. A meta-analysis published in 2020 revealed that mindfulness could become a practical psychological resource for caregivers taking care of their relatives with dementia.

- **Accept help**: It is a great idea to list some ways other people can help you and let the person willing to help you choose what they would like to do. For example, a friend can offer to help you take your loved one with dementia for a 15-minute walk a couple of times a week. Alternatively, you can allow a family member to run an errand on your behalf, such as shopping for groceries or cooking for you.
- **Outsource caregiving responsibilities**: If you can outsource caregiving responsibilities, do just that. There are assisted living facilities, adult day care centers, and home health services that are options worth exploring. Alternatively, getting an extra caregiver can be helpful, and you will have more time to spend with family or even enjoy the time you spend with your loved one with dementia because you will not have to be helping them or always be on all the time.
- **Set realistic goals**: Break down large tasks into smaller, practical steps that you can do one at a time. Smaller steps become easy mountains to climb to reach the top of the mountain where your large tasks are completed and you feel accomplished. Prioritize

making lists and establishing a daily routine. Learn to say no to things that will drain you, such as hosting dinner.

- **Set personal health goals**: For example, it is crucial to get good quality sleep. So, you can set goals to ensure you develop a good sleep routine. Also, you will expand your goals to thinking about what time in the day is best for you to be physically active at least three days or more in a week. There are other goals to consider, such as eating a healthy diet and drinking plenty of water.

- **Take something off your plate**: Learn to delegate or postpone that can help. A review published in 2018 revealed that paying close attention to lessening the burden of caregiving, such as reducing work hours, paying for extra caregivers, and lowering expectations of your loved one with dementia, is more helpful than emotion-focused coping, including avoidance or wishful thinking.

- **Join a support group**: Finding a community of caregivers you can relate with on different levels is helpful. Talking to other people about your struggles and asking them how they handle certain situations you experience can be extremely helpful for you to connect with people who are or were in similar situations. It can help you get through challenging times.

- **Permit yourself to feel what you are going through**: You may have normal negative emotions that do not mean you are a horrible person. On the contrary, being a caregiver, there is this misconception that you must always be strong for your loved one and that crying is a sign of weakness. It is crucial to allow yourself to feel what you are going through and not suppress your emotions. In other words, be strong in front of your loved one with dementia, but behind closed doors, allow yourself to cry or feel whatever emotions you are experiencing.
- **See a therapist**: Seeking mental health support from a qualified mental health practitioner can help you manage the stresses that come with caregiving. It can help immensely when you are already burned out or about to get burned out. Also, unexpected life circumstances can arise, such as a family member's death, which can add to your plate of emotions that you need to deal with a counselor.
- **Maintain your relationships**: Do not forget that you are someone's spouse or child beyond your caregiving role, and it is important not to abandon that role for whatever reason. If you are a daughter or a son to your parents, spend time with them; have dinner with them. Be present with your family when you are with them, and be the daughter or son your parents know you to be.

- **Practice a preferred relaxation technique**: To combat the stress that comes with taking care of a loved one with dementia, you can engage in relaxation techniques, such as deep breathing exercises, meditation, or yoga. It will help to boost your energy levels and improve your mood, which will help with activating your body's natural relaxation response.
- **Talk to someone**: Talk to someone that you trust, whether they are a friend, family member, or therapist, about what you are experiencing in your life. It can be highly cathartic and a great stress reliever to talk to someone face-to-face and have them listen to your frustrations and grievances.
- **Exercise**: Regular exercise is vital to keep you physically fit and mentally well, as it helps you release endorphins that can improve your mood. You can aim for at least 30 minutes to exercise for most days of the week. If you cannot commit to 30 minutes at one time, consider breaking it into 10-minute sessions throughout the day.
- **Attend your regular medical checkups**: Visit your medical doctor regularly for checkups and pay attention to the signs and symptoms of excessive stress. It is best not to let go of the people and activities that you love when you are burdened with caregiving to help maintain your health and peace of mind when you do so. Take time away from

caregiving to spend time with your friends and family and pursue your hobbies and interests that bring enjoyment.
- **Eat well**: Ensuring you learn and practice healthy eating habits like the Mediterranean diet is excellent for overall health and can help nourish the brain. Invest in trying new recipes that contain relatively small amounts of meat, more colorful fruits and vegetables, and good fats, such as olive oil, and involve your loved one with dementia.
- **Practice acceptance**: When faced with the unfairness or burden of caregiving for a loved one's health condition, there is often this sense of wanting to understand the situation and asking yourself why this is happening. Nonetheless, you can spend a lot of time and energy dwelling on matters that are out of your control and for which there are no specific, straightforward answers. Also, you will not feel any better doing this to yourself. It is better to avoid feeling sorry for yourself or wanting to blame someone else.
- **Embrace your decision to care for your loved one with dementia**: Tell yourself that regardless of any resentments or how burdened you may feel, you have chosen to care for your loved one with dementia consciously. Focus on the positive reasons that informed your decision. For example, you decided to care for your loved one to repay your

parents with dementia for taking care of you growing up, or it could be because of your values or role-modeling behavior that you want your children to follow. These meaningful motivations can help you keep going in tough times.

- **Look on the bright side**: Consider the different ways caregiving has positively changed you or brought you closer to the loved one you are taking care of or to other relatives.
- **Do not let caregiving take over your life**: Because it is easier to accept challenging situations when other areas of a person's life are rewarding, it is vital not to let caregiving become your entire existence. Spend your time and energy doing purposeful things that give you meaning, whether it is your children, family, or career.
- **Focus your mind on the things in your control**: There is no way to add more hours in a day, or you may be unable to force any of your relatives to help you out more. Rather than concern yourself with things that are out of your control, it would be better to focus on how you react to problems as they come because that is something you can control.
- **Celebrate the small wins**: If you begin to feel discouraged, take some time to remind yourself of all the hard work you have put in to take good care of your loved one. You do not need to cure your loved one's mental health condition to feel you have made

a difference in their life. Do not underestimate how vital it is to make your loved one with dementia feel safe, secure, comfortable, and cherished.

SUMMARY

- Taking care of yourself is similar to taking an oxygen mask in the case of an emergency on an airplane. It will be difficult for you to take care of anyone else when you have not taken care of yourself first. It is never a selfish act to do some self-care every day, even if it is for 5 minutes every day.
- Caregiver burnout is feeling physically, emotionally, and mentally exhausted from taking on too many caregiving responsibilities for an extended period.
- The symptoms of caregiver burnout can range from noticing changes in attitude, from feeling love to feeling negative and not caring anymore, feeling crabby, losing interest in things you previously enjoyed, noticing changes in eating and sleeping patterns and experiencing weight loss. Furthermore, getting sick often and getting irritated easily.
- There were numerous tips suggested on how to manage caregiver burnout. All the tips have a couple of things in common: It is crucial to set time to focus on maintaining your social and family relationships and take time to take care of your mental, physical, and emotional health through therapy, relaxation

techniques, exercising, and regular visits to the doctor, accepting what you can control and what you cannot control, and celebrating yourself through it all.

Discussing self-care in the book's last chapter does not mean you must be last. Understandably, you may see yourself as the least priority, but you must also remember that taking care of yourself is not selfish. After all, if you do not take care of yourself, how can you provide quality care for your loved one with dementia?

CONCLUSION

The mind of a person with dementia is like a "silent thief" because the brain damage negatively affects their cognitive functioning and robs a person of who they are, the memories they have made in their life, and their sense of control. Dementia is a disease that is terrifying to many people, but yet it needs to be understood to manage this fear. It has many symptoms and underlying causes for developing the mental health condition. There are many misconceptions about dementia, and one of those that have been disputed is that dementia is synonymous with Alzheimer's disease. There are about five types of dementia. At least, when you hear someone talking about dementia, you will immediately think of more than one type of dementia and the different stages of dementia. Learning about the different types and stages of dementia helps determine the best care for your loved one with dementia.

The various types of dementia have some similarities in presenting symptoms, especially in the early stages of dementia. However, the disease's impact on the brain can affect a person's thinking, executive functioning, emotions, behavior, speech, language, perception, and relationships. Learning to cope with the prognosis of dementia can be distressing for both the person diagnosed with it and those who care for them. It can lead the caregiver and the person's loved ones to their breaking point. Nonetheless, there are effective techniques to combat the negative impact of dementia and control the symptoms to have some normalcy and maintain relationships. Communication is one of those effective techniques.

Being equipped with different ways to communicate with your loved one with dementia can help to manage situations whereby they have difficulty finding the right words to say, which is a consequence of the memory loss they experience. Several simple and practical tips were suggested to help with managing memory problems. It can be challenging to deal with memory loss in the middle to late stages of dementia. Nonetheless, empowering yourself with strategies and skills to cope with it can lessen the burden of dealing with memory loss and behavioral changes.

Surviving the struggles that come with the behavioral changes your loved one experiences due to dementia is never easy. Getting adequate knowledge and support can make it more manageable, as well as other aspects of their lives, such as bathing, exercising, and eating. Helping them maintain their physical health and well-being is not always a struggle, but it can be fun. Several activities were presented that can benefit both of you by doing things you enjoy that can boost your relationship.

Committing to doing simple activities together can benefit your mental and physical health and deepen your connection with each other while dealing with dementia. The suggested activities are designed to do precisely that. After all, caregiving can be stressful and exhausting at times. Learning the importance of self-care can only help keep your health and well-being intact.

Trying out different self-care techniques can help you determine what works for you. Also, it can help you to avoid that dreadful caregiver burnout. Taking care of yourself does not mean you only care about your health and well-being above your loved one with dementia all the time, but it does mean that you recognize that you are a priority. Self-care is like performing a selfless act of caring for yourself every day, even for five minutes. When you do that regularly, the quality of care you provide to your loved one with dementia will remain consistently positive.

REFERENCES

Agespace. (n.d.). *8 Practical Tips to Help Someone With Dementia to Eat More.* Agespace. https://www.agespace.org/dementia/tips-to-help-someone-with-dementia-to-eat-more

Alzheimer's Research UK. (November, 2021). *What Happens to Someone With Dementia?* Alzheimer's Research UK. https://www.alzheimersresearchuk.org/kids/juniors/what-is-dementia/what-happens-to-someone-with-dementia/

Alzheimer's Association. (2023a). *Brain Facts.* Alzheimer's Association. https://www.alz.org/help-support/resources/kids-teens/brain-facts

Alzheimer's Association. (2023b). *Alzheimer's Disease Facts and Figures.* Alzheimer's Association. https://www.alz.org/alzheimers-dementia/facts-figures

Alzheimer's Association. (n.d.a). *Stages of Alzheimer's.* Alzheimer's Association. https://www.alz.org/alzheimers-dementia/stages

Alzheimer's Association. (n.d.b). *Communication and Alzheimer's.* Alzheimer's Association. https://www.alz.org/help-support/caregiving/daily-care/communications

Alzheimer's Association. (n.d.c). *Memory Loss and Confusion.* Alzheimer's Association. https://www.alz.org/help-support/caregiving/stages-behaviors/memory-loss-confusion

Alzheimer's Association. (n.d.d). *Medications for Memory, Cognition and Dementia-Related Behaviors.* Alzheimer's Association. https://www.alz.org/alzheimers-dementia/treatments/medications-for-memory

Alzheimer's Association. (n.d.e). *Stages and Behaviors.* Alzheimer's Association. https://www.alz.org/help-support/caregiving/stages-behaviors

Alzheimer's Association. (n.d.f). *Food and Eating.* Alzheimer's Association. https://www.alz.org/help-support/caregiving/daily-care/food-eating

Alzheimer's Association. (n.d.g). *Personal Care.* Alzheimer's Association. https://www.alz.org/national/documents/brochure_personalcare.pdf

Alzheimer's Association. (n.d.h). *Be a Healthy Caregiver.* Alzheimer's

Association. https://www.alz.org/help-support/caregiving/caregiver-health/be_a_healthy_caregiver

ADI. (n.d.a). *Find Local Support.* Alzheimer's Disease International. https://www.alzint.org/about/find-local-support/

ADI. (n.d.b). *Symptoms of Dementia.* Alzheimer's Disease International. https://www.alzint.org/about/symptoms-of-dementia/

Alzheimer's Society. (February 24, 2021a). *The Progression, Signs and Stages of Dementia.* Alzheimer's Society. https://www.alzheimers.org.uk/about-dementia/symptoms-and-diagnosis/how-dementia-progresses/progression-stages-dementia

Alzheimer's Society. (September 01, 2021b). *Dementia With Lewy Bodies: What Is It And What Causes It?* Alzheimer's Society. https://www.alzheimers.org.uk/about-dementia/types-dementia/dementia-with-lewy-bodies

Alzheimer's Society. (August 11, 2021c). *Memory Aids and Tools.* Alzheimer's Society. https://www.alzheimers.org.uk/get-support/staying-independent/memory-aids-and-tools

Alzheimer's Society. (September 02, 2021d). *How to Support a Person With Dementia to Wash, Bathe and Shower.* Alzheimer's Society. https://www.alzheimers.org.uk/get-support/daily-living/washing-bathing-showering-tips

Alzheimer's Society. (March 08, 2021e). *How to Support a Person With Dementia to get Dressed or Change Clothes.* Alzheimer's Society. https://www.alzheimers.org.uk/get-support/daily-living/getting-dressed-changing-clothes#content-start

Alzheimer's Society. (June 21, 2022a). *Symptoms of Vascular Dementia.* Alzheimer's Society. https://www.alzheimers.org.uk/about-dementia/types-dementia/symptoms-vascular-dementia#content-start

Alzheimer's Society. (June 27, 2022b). *Understanding and Supporting a Person With Dementia.* Alzheimer's Society. https://www.alzheimers.org.uk/get-support/help-dementia-care/understanding-supporting-person-dementia

Alzheimer's Society. (April 13, 2023). *Alzheimer's Disease.* Alzheimer's Society. https://www.alzheimers.org.uk/about-dementia/types-dementia/alzheimers-disease

Alzheimer's Society. (n.d.a.). *Frontotemporal Dementia.* Alzheimer's Society. https://www.alzheimers.org.uk/about-dementia/types-dementia/frontotemporal-dementia

Alzheimer's Society. (n.d.b.). *Exercise in the Early to Middle Stages of Dementia.* Alzheimer's Society. https://www.alzheimers.org.uk/get-support/daily-living/exercise/early-middle-dementia

Alzheimer's Society. (n.d.c). *Exercise in the Later Stages of Dementia.* Alzheimer's Society. https://www.alzheimers.org.uk/get-support/daily-living/exercise-later-stages

Alzheimer Society of Canada. (n.d.). *Understanding How Your Relationship May Change.* Alzheimer Society of Canada. https://alzheimer.ca/en/help-support/i-have-friend-or-family-member-who-lives-dementia/understanding-how-your-relationship

Az. (June 06, 2017). *The Silent Thief.* Medium. https://medium.com/@sandraaz/the-silent-thief-2d742120616a

Being Patient. (n.d.). *How Gadgets Can Help People Live With Dementia.* Being Patient. https://www.beingpatient.com/assistive-technology-dementia/

Better Health. (May 31, 2014a). *Dementia - Behavioral Changes.* Better Health. https://www.betterhealth.vic.gov.au/health/conditionsandtreatments/dementia-behaviour-changes#sundowning-in-dementia

Better Health. (May 31, 2014b). *Dementia - Emotional Changes.* Better Health. https://www.betterhealth.vic.gov.au/health/conditionsandtreatments/dementia-emotional-changes

Better Health. (May 31, 2014c). *Dementia - Hygiene.* Better Health. https://www.betterhealth.vic.gov.au/health/conditionsandtreatments/dementia-hygiene

Britton, B. (n.d.). *The Emotional Impact of Dementia.* Elder. https://www.elder.org/the-elder/the-emotional-impact-of-dementia/

CarePredict. (May 23, 2018). *What Does Dementia Feel Like?* CarePredict. https://www.carepredict.com/blog/neuroscientist-experiences-dementia-symptoms/

Centers for Disease Control and Prevention. (April 5, 2019). *About Dementia.* Centers for Disease Control and Prevention. https://www.cdc.gov/aging/dementia/index.html

Cleveland Clinic. (January 13, 2019). *Caregiver Burnout.* Cleveland Clinic. https://my.clevelandclinic.org/health/diseases/9225-caregiver-burnout

Clayton, T. (December 05, 2017). *Tracey's Story: 'Caring for a Person With Dementia Can Be All-Consuming'.* Alzheimer's Society. https://www.alzheimers.org.uk/alzheimers-society-blog/traceys-story-caring-person-dementia-can-be-all-consuming

Cohen, M. (January 28, 2022). *How to Avoid Caregiver Burnout, According to Experts that Understand the Signs.* Prevention. https://www.prevention.com/health/a36173944/what-is-caregiver-burnout/

Conolly, P. (July 30, 2016). *Dementia; Dreadful Any Dya of the Week.* Pauline Conolly. https://paulineconolly.com/2016/dementia/

Craig, S. (September 08, 2021). *Helpful Daily Activities for Dementia Patients: 50 Expert Tips and Suggestions to Keep Your Loved One Engaged.* Careforth Blog. https://www.careforth.com/blog/helpful-daily-activities-for-dementia-patients-50-expert-tips-and-suggestions-to-keep-your-loved-one-engaged

Crystal Run Healthcare. (April 16, 2019). *Alzheimer's and Dementia: Which Areas of the Brain Are Affected?* Crystal Run Healthcare. https://www.crystalrunhealthcare.com/articles/what-areas-of-the-brain-are-affected-by-alzheimers-and-dementia

DailyCaring Editorial Team. (n.d.a). *3 Stages of Dementia: What to Expect as the Disease Progresses.* DailyCaring. https://dailycaring.com/3-stages-of-dementia-what-to-expect/

DailyCaring Editorial Team. (n.d.b). *How to Talk to Someone With Dementia: Calm, Positive Body Language.* DailyCaring. https://dailycaring.com/dementia-communication-techniques-calm-positive-body-language/

Dayton, C. (March 18, 2021). *Guide to Caring for a Parent With Dementia at Home.* Salus. https://www.salushomecare.com/blog/caring-for-a-parent-with-dementia-at-home/

Dementia Australia. (2016). *Mental Exercise and Dementia.* Dementia Australia. https://www.dementia.org.au/sites/default/files/helpsheets/Helpsheet-DementiaQandA06-MentalExercise_english.pdf

Dementia Care Central. (January 26, 2023). *Stages of Alzheimer's & Dementia: Durations & Scales Used to Measure Progression (GDS, FAST & CDR).* Dementia Care Central. https://www.dementiacarecentral.com/aboutdementia/facts/stages/

DementiaUK. (August 2020). *The Emotional Impact of a Dementia Diagnosis.* DementiaUK. https://www.dementiauk.org/get-support/understanding-changes-in-dementia/emotional-impact-of-the-diagnosis/#impact

Family Advisory Board of the Transitions ACR. (2019). *For Families or Caregivers:*

Self-Care is Putting on YOUR Oxygen Mask First. Family Advisory Board of the Transitions ACR. https://repository.escholarship.umassmed.edu/bitstream/handle/20.500.14038/44258/Self_Care_is_Putting_on_YOUR_Oxygen_Mask_First_w_attribution_12.9.19.pdf?sequence=3&isAllowed=y

Frontier Management. (n.d.). *How to Recognize Dementia in Seniors.* Frontier Management. https://frontiermgmt.com/blog/how-to-recognize-dementia-in-seniors/

Greenwald, M. (June 28, 2018). *35 Crazy Facts About Your Memory.* Best Life. https://bestlifeonline.com/facts-about-memory/

Gregory, A. & Geddes, L. (September 21, 2021). *More Than 41M Dementia Cases Globally Are Undiagnosed - Study.* The Guardian. https://www.theguardian.com/society/2021/sep/21/more-than-41m-dementia-cases-globally-are-undiagnosed-study

Gupta, S. (August 01, 2022). *Symptoms of Alzheimer's Disease.* Very Well Mind. https://www.verywellmind.com/alzheimer-s-disease-signs-symptoms-and-comorbidities-5190167

Heerema, E. (January 25, 2020). *Eating, Appetite Changes and Weight Loss in Dementia.* Very Well Health. https://www.verywellhealth.com/eating-appetite-changes-and-weight-loss-in-dementia-98582

Heerema, E. (August 31, 2021a). *Frontotemporal Dementia Overview.* Very Well Mind. https://www.verywellhealth.com/what-is-frontotemporal-dementia-98747

Heerema, E. (September 26, 2021b). *Mixed Dementia and Its Symptoms.* Very Well Health. https://www.verywellhealth.com/what-is-mixed-dementia-98748

Herndon, J. (February 07, 2022). *Everything You Need to Know About Alzheimer's Disease.* Healthline. https://www.healthline.com/health/alzheimers-disease

Hill, C. (July 26, 2022a). *What Is Vascular Dementia?* Very Well Health. https://www.verywellhealth.com/vascular-dementia-98802#toc-vascular-dementia-symptoms

Hill, C. (March 31, 2022b). *Overview of Lewy body Dementia.* Very Well Mind. https://www.verywellhealth.com/brain-syndrome-dementia-lewy-bodies-98801#toc-symptoms

Hill, C. (April 23, 2022c). *How to Still Eat Well in Late-Stage Alzheimer's Disease.*

Very Well Health. https://www.verywellhealth.com/enhancing-nutrition-in-late-stage-alzheimers-disease-97761

Hobson, G. (May 09, 2023). *Dealing With Dementia Behaviors: Tips for Understanding and Coping.* A Place for Mom. https://www.aplaceformom.com/caregiver-resources/articles/dementia-behaviors

Holland, K. (February 14, 2022). *What Is Vascular Dementia?* Healthline. https://www.alzheimers.org.uk/about-dementia/types-dementia/symptoms-vascular-dementia#content-start

Holland, K. (March 31, 2017). *Frontotemporal Dementia.* Healthline. https://www.healthline.com/health/frontotemporal-dementia

IMDb. (n.d.). *Evelyn Keyes Biography.* IMDb. https://www.imdb.com/name/nm0450810/bio

IMDb. (n.d.). *Robin Williams (1951 - 2014).* IMDb. https://www.imdb.com/name/nm0000245/

Ivy Palmer Live-in Care Services. (n.d.). *What Are The 7 Stages of Dementia?* Ivy Palmer Live-in Care Services. https://www.ip-live-in-care.co.uk/7-stages-dementia/

Johns Hopkins Medical Institutions. (July 23, 2009). *"Close Caregiver Relationship May Slow Alzheimer's Decline."* Science Daily. https://www.sciencedaily.com/releases/2009/07/090722191219.htm

Kennard, C. (January 29, 2023). *Famous People With Alzheimer's Disease or Dementia.* Verywell Health. https://www.verywellhealth.com/famous-people-with-alzheimers-98082

Lawler, M. (March 29, 2023). *Caregiver Burnout: What It Is, Signs You're Experiencing It and How to Cope.* Everyday Health. https://www.everydayhealth.com/burnout/caregiver-burnout/

Leonard, W. (February 11, 2022). *Everything to Know About Dementia.* Healthline. https://www.healthline.com/health/dementia

Leung, W. (April 2, 2019). *'There's hope.'Princess Yasmin Aga Khan opens up about her mother Rita Hayworth and Alzheimer's disease.* The Globe and Mail. https://www.theglobeandmail.com/life/health-and-fitness/article-princess-yasmin-aga-khan-discusses-her-mother-rita-hayworth-and/

London, B. (November 16, 2020). *Do's and Don'ts for Communicating With Someone Who Has Dementia.* Bayada. https://blog.bayada.com/be-healthy/dos-and-donts-for-communicating-with-someone-who-has-dementia

Long Island Alzheimer's and Dementia Center. (May 13, 2021). *Celebrities with dementia*. Long Island Alzheimer's and Dementia Center. https://www.lidementia.org/celebrities-with-dementia/

Long Island Alzheimer's and Dementia Center. (2023). *Lewy Body Dementia*. Long Island Alzheimer's and Dementia Center. https://www.lidementia.org/alzheimers-disease/types-of-dementia/lewy-body-dementia/

MacGill, M. (April 19, 2023). *What Is Dementia? Symptoms, Stages, Types and More*. Medical News Today. https://www.medicalnewstoday.com/articles/142214

Mayo Clinic. (March 22, 2022). *Caregiver Stress: Tips for Taking Care of Yourself*. Mayo Clinic. https://www.mayoclinic.org/healthy-lifestyle/stress-management/in-depth/caregiver-stress/art-20044784

Microsoft Start. (n.d.). *Ask the Professionals*. Microsoft Start. https://microsoftstart.msn.com/en-za/health/ask-professionals/dysphagia?questionid=fz9wawkx&type=condition&ocid=entnewsntp&source=bingmainline_conditionqna

National Foundation of Swallowing Disorders. (July 02, 2017). *Caregiver's Guide to Dysphagia in Dementia*. National Foundation of Swallowing Disorders. https://swallowingdisorderfoundation.com/caregivers-guide-dysphagia-dementia/

National Health System [NHS]. (February 13, 2023). *Communicating With Someone With Dementia*. National Health System. https://www.nhs.uk/conditions/dementia/communication-and-dementia/

National Institute on Aging. (May 18, 2017). *Bathing, Dressing, and Grooming: Alzheimer's Caregiving Tips*. National Institute on Aging. https://www.nia.nih.gov/health/bathing-dressing-and-grooming-alzheimers-caregiving-tips

National Institute on Aging. (n.d.). *Tips for Caregivers and Families of People With Dementia*. National Institute on Aging. https://www.alzheimers.gov/life-with-dementia/tips-caregivers

Nehring, A. (June 03, 2016). *Alzheimer's: A Real Love Story ...* Alzheimer's Association. https://www.alz.org/blog/alz/june_2016/alzheimer_s_a_real_love_story%E2%80%A6

NHS. (January 04, 2021). *Coping With Dementia Behavior Changes*. National Health System. https://www.nhs.uk/conditions/dementia/behaviour/

OurParents Staff. (April 20, 2023). *Love and Dementia: How to Support a Couple Coping With Memory Loss*. OurParents. https://www.ourparents.com/

senior-health/coping-with-memory-loss

Pallardy, R. (October 17, 2022). *Ben Bradlee.* Britannica. https://www.britannica.com/biography/Benjamin-C-Bradlee

Pietrangelo, A. (January 20, 2022). *Everything You Need to Know About Lewy Body Dementia.* Healthline. https://www.healthline.com/health/dementia/lewy-body-dementia

Poncela-Casasnovas, J., Gutiérrez-Roig, M., Gracia-Lázaro, C., Vicens, J., Gómez-Gardeñes, J., Perelló, J., ... & Sánchez, A. (2016). Humans display a reduced set of consistent behavioral phenotypes in dyadic games. *Science advances, 2*(8), e1600451.

Robinson, L., Wayne, M., & Segal, J. (February 23, 2023). *Alzheimer's and Dementia Care: Help for Family Caregivers.* HelpGuide. https://www.helpguide.org/articles/alzheimers-dementia-aging/tips-for-alzheimers-caregivers.htm

Samuels, C. (May 09, 2023). *20 Engaging Activities for People With Dementia at Home.* A Place for Mom. https://www.aplaceformom.com/caregiver-resources/articles/dementia-activities

Senior Services of America. (2022). *Meaningful Activities for Dementia Patients: 15 Ways to Keep Your Loved One Engaged.* Senior Services of America. https://seniorservicesofamerica.com/blog/15-meaningful-activities-for-dementia-patients/

Simple English Wikipedia. (October 21, 2022). *Pauline Phillips.* Simple Wikipedia. https://simple.wikipedia.org/wiki/Pauline_Phillips#cite_note-New_York_Times-1

Smith, M., Segal, J., & White M. (February 23, 2023). *Alzheimer's and Dementia Behavior Management.* HelpGuide. https://www.helpguide.org/articles/alzheimers-dementia-aging/alzheimers-behavior-management.htm

Smith, M. (February 24, 2023). *Caregiver Stress and Burnout.* HelpGuide. https://www.helpguide.org/articles/stress/caregiver-stress-and-burnout.htm

Sports Reference. (April 16, 2023). *Marv Owen.* Baseball Reference. https://www.baseball-reference.com/players/o/owenma01.shtml

Sports Reference. (April 16, 2023). *Bill Quackenbush.* Hockey Reference. https://www.hockey-reference.com/players/q/quackbi01.html

Sports Reference. (2016). *Betty Robinson.* Sports Reference. https://web.

archive.org/web/20200417173344/https://www.sports-reference.com/olympics/athletes/ro/betty-robinson-1.html

Stringfellow, A. (March 20, 2019). *Activities for Dementia Patients: 50 Tips and Ideas to Keep Patients With Dementia Engaged.* Careforth Blog. https://www.careforth.com/blog/activities-for-dementia-patients-50-tips-and-ideas-to-keep-patients-with-dementia-engaged

Stuart, A. (November 27, 2020). *Brain Exercises and Dementia.* WebMD. https://www.webmd.com/alzheimers/guide/preventing-dementia-brain-exercises

The Editors of Encyclopaedia Britannica. (January 22, 2023). *A.E. Van Vogt.* Britannica. https://www.britannica.com/biography/A-E-Van-Vogt

The Editors of Encyclopaedia Britannica. (November 12, 2022). *Burgess Meredith.* Britannica. https://www.britannica.com/biography/Burgess-Meredith

The Editors of Encyclopaedia Britannica. (March 7, 2023). *Harold Wilson.* Britannica. https://www.britannica.com/biography/Harold-Wilson-Baron-Wilson-of-Rievaulx

The Editors of Encyclopaedia Britannica. (April 7, 2023). *Ronald Reagan.* Britannica. https://www.britannica.com/biography/Ronald-Reagan

The Editors of Encyclopaedia Britannica. (April 7, 2023). *Rosa Parks.* Britannica. https://www.britannica.com/biography/Rosa-Parks

The Editors of Encyclopaedia Britannica. (April 7, 2023). *Sean Connery.* Britannica. https://www.britannica.com/biography/Sean-Connery

The Editors of Encyclopaedia Britannica. (April 8, 2023). *Sugar Ray Robinson.* Britannica. https://www.britannica.com/sports/Golden-Gloves

The Editors of Encyclopaedia Britannica. (April 10, 2022). *Iris Murdoch.* Britannica. https://www.britannica.com/biography/Iris-Murdoch

Tikkanen, A. (January 27, 2023). *Pat Summitt.* Britannica. https://www.britannica.com/biography/Pat-Summitt

Vera. (2023). *What Effects Does Dementia Have on the Brain?* Vera. https://www.veramusic.com/blog/what-effects-does-dementia-have-on-the-brain

WebMD. (February 08, 2023). *Dementia.* WebMD. https://www.webmd.com/alzheimers/types-dementia

WebMD Editorial Contributors. (November 27, 2022). *When Someone With Alzheimer's Won't Eat or Drink.* WebMD. https://www.webmd.com/alzheimers/not-eating-drinking-alzheimers

Wikipedia, The Free Encyclopedia. (February 1, 2023). *Raul Silva Henriquez.* Wikipedia, The Free Encyclopedia. https://en.wikipedia.org/wiki/Ra%C3%BAl_Silva_Henr%C3%ADquez#cite_note-1

Williams, S. S. (2016). The Terrorist Inside My Husband's Brain. Neurology. *87*(13). 1308 - 1311. doi: 10.1212/WNL.0000000000003162

World Health Organization [WHO]. (2023, March 15). *Dementia.* World Health Organization. https://www.who.int/news-room/fact-sheets/detail/dementia

Young, H. (April 4, 2023). *Margaret Thatcher.* Britannica. https://www.britannica.com/biography/Margaret-Thatcher